T0132277

SLEEP
STRENGTH

CLAES ZELL

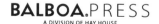
BALBOA.PRESS
A DIVISION OF HAY HOUSE

Balboa Press books may be ordered through booksellers or by contacting:

Balboa Press
A Division of Hay House
1663 Liberty Drive
Bloomington, IN 47403
www.balboapress.com
1 (877) 407-4847

Because of the dynamic nature of the Internet, any web addresses or links contained in this book may have changed since publication and may no longer be valid. The views expressed in this work are solely those of the author and do not necessarily reflect the views of the publisher, and the publisher hereby disclaims any responsibility for them.

The author of this book does not dispense medical advice or prescribe the use of any technique as a form of treatment for physical, emotional, or medical problems without the advice of a physician, either directly or indirectly. The intent of the author is only to offer information of a general nature to help you in your quest for emotional and spiritual well-being. In the event you use any of the information in this book for yourself, which is your constitutional right, the author and the publisher assume no responsibility for your actions.

Any people depicted in stock imagery provided by Getty Images are models, and such images are being used for illustrative purposes only.
Certain stock imagery © Getty Images.

Print information available on the last page.

ISBN: 978-1-9822-4341-8 (sc)
ISBN: 978-1-9822-4342-5 (e)

Balboa Press rev. date: 02/29/2020

Claes!

You have kept me awake late with your outstanding educational and extremely well written book. What tremendous research work you put in to successfully convey the latest findings. I have carefully read your book from cover to cover amazed and impressed by your knowledge. Also, grateful and touched on the mention on the thanks page.

Josefin E

Acknowledgment

A huge thanks to my brother **Peter**, who read the script indefinitely and provided valuable tips and advice to improve the content.

An equally big thanks to **Friskis & Svettis**, F&S, established as a non-profit organization in Stockholm (98 000 members) in 1978 to promote an Active lifestyle through fun, high quality, affordable workout classes. Now also operates outside Sweden.

Maria Olsson, Plant Manager F&S Gärdet, who helps me with illustrations. **Josefin Engfelt**, PR & Editor, who supported me and showed great interest with planned lectures within the organization.

Contents

Foreword

In my first book I describe my long experience of stretching techniques to make the body relaxed, alpha rhythm. I started preparing for a follow-up to show more relaxing techniques than stretching, but fate wanted me to go a different direction. A way that initially seems to be a contradiction to what I have taught earlier.

Fate was further strengthened, and I got to experience in real time what I write about in this book, neither more nor less. At the end of the text of this script, I was reminded that much can happen in an instant, a small accident and my right foot got plastered. It was a big change for me who usually practice 4-5 times a week right across the street where I live.

For some reason, higher powers wanted me to know what happens when the body is not activated. Played football in Stockholm as a youth and continued with judo training for 14 years, which resulted in a participation in the Swedish Championship. For a period, I started to run and participated in Stockholm marathon. But I felt that I still wanted to build muscles and not just wear running. I started at Rellos Gym near KTH (Royal Institute of Technology), where I was studying at that time, in -79. Almost half century of regular training.

An additional problem arose more and more and which became acute - sleep began to break. Sleep - my topic for ten years since I started writing my first English edition. Funny, or not, that's what I started writing about in this book, muscle wasting. The leg muscles begin to think with a furious pace, mainly in the plastered leg. I had lost surprisingly much in six weeks. The muscles disappeared quickly, so as my sleep quality, although, my sleep quality at that time had a quite complex medical reasons due to rehabilitation program.

What a lesson hasn't this period in my life been. Keeping up with fitness and strength training, in order to achieve a reserve power for future hardships is something good for everyone. There is much to think about in today's hectic society, but training constitutes a basic bolt for the vast majority of people to cope with the pressure of a modern society.

This book describes what a combination of muscle types interacts with sleep ability. Many people sleep well, but how is it possible that some people fall asleep immediately and others climbing on the walls. There must be something natural for the sleep group that makes the good sleep possible. Of course, your heritages make a lot of how you sleep. But one can learn a lot only by studying "the good sleepers", in order to overcome bad genes, some effort may be needed, but it can be worthwhile.

My knowledge of topics has made me search and read thousands of reports and just as many hours of stubborn work to seek clues, to sew my muscle / sleep theory together. Helping people to improve their ability to relax, to sleep deeper, or not to wake up during the night can be difficult to achieve. But doing this in a natural way without sleep medicine has from the beginning been my ultimate goal.

With this book, I give you these specific keys - the muscles, to overcome the signs of insomnia. With scientific reports, I want to reinforce my assumptions, but the sleep problem has many faces and may therefore need other measures for some people. However, there is nothing to prevent supplementing my keys with other appropriate measures that can help individuals in need. Give my exercises the chance for you, to turn bad sleep into something better and which means that you may discover - the holy grail of sleep. Stay on my sleep trip.

Good Luck and Good Night!

Stockholm Feb 2020
Claes Zell

Introduction

The topic - muscle strength has been found in many medical reports in recent years and mostly to complement older people. Strong muscles make daily life more achievable, independence longer in life, and especially for men who lose 1-2% of the hormone testosterone from the middle age.

The testosterone has many important functions and maintaining training of the strong muscle types drives testosterone production. It is so easy to give up training or an active life when you get older. After a long active life with jobs and social interaction, then when the pension is suddenly imminent, you just want to take it easy. It's okay for a period, but not too long. Continuing an active life is important for maintaining or pumping up the body systems. Exercise makes the body smooth, like oil in an engine

Since the 90's there have been many relaxation programs for the common man to buy. Sitting relaxed, listening to music and a quiet voice that brings you down in a relaxing state, was the great message to stressful fellow human beings. Absolutely no bad message, but it is quite difficult to mentally relax with body full of tense muscles.

However, there is much to learn from ancient wisdom, especially by looking a little at Eastern tradition. Both Indian and Chinese medical theories have archetypes, constitutions since eons for the strong sleepers and the weak.

All people are different, but have similarities. I usually describe differences between people's ability to sleep by referring to a meeting and a dialogue with a friend, about my book projects in the subject of sleep. In the writing of my first book, I talked to a friend and said: I work with a book on sleep and sleep problems. It became a moment of silence, and then the question came, why? He had no idea why a book was needed to be written. Take a deep breath, put your head on a pillow, relax and sleep, he said with a very confident voice. For many people, it is just that, nothing to think about, just relax and soon you are in your dream land. Unfortunately, consensus among the public says another story, it's not that easy. If you have no idea or interest in your own sleep, you probably get enough sleep hours. But for a bunch of people, 30 plus percent, I wrote this second Swedish book.

A good sleep is crucial for many medical parameters and if deep sleep is maintained without any sleep medication, it is worth a lot. It's not just about health. A Swedish study shows that the facial region is an important part of the communication between people. Insomnia can reduce or affect your chances of a good career due to less healthy appearance. The study examined the facial signals that show when someone lacks sleep. Lack of sleep is recognized by more hanging eyelids, red and swollen eyes, more wrinkles and finer lines. Everyone wants to show off their very best, look fresh, but it is most difficult to achieve when good sleep does not occur.

Insomnia can also be devastating overall, since acute sleep deprivation can be linked to brain damage according to another Swedish study. The study investigates whether total sleep stability affects circulating concentrations of specific neurons and proteins in humans. The researchers suggest that increased concentration may indicate neuronal damage due to lack of sleep time. After a lack of sleep for a long time, many steps take the help of sleeping pills to sleep. Sleep medicine is common throughout the world, but it is hardly a solution for a long time. The use of benzodiazepines to treat insomnia increases the risk of Alzheimer's disease. A study of nearly 9,000 elderly subjects showed that the risk of Alzheimer's disease was increased up to 51% in those who had used benzodiazepines over the past 5 years. The use of benzodiazepines increased the risk at 6 months or longer. Our results are of great importance to public health, especially considering the use of the elderly and the increased incidence of dementia in developed countries, the researchers wrote.

The easily observable effects of sleep in everyday life are not surprising that there has been scientific interest in sleep. Sleep epidemiology has a recognizable history of just over three decades, but it is still found that obesity and smoking give 5-6 times more hits in scientific publications. However, sleep-related research is rapidly increasing.

Epidemiological studies show that it is not good to sleep too long. Studies that assessed sleep duration and mortality showed that both those who had too short a bedtime and too long had an increased risk of premature death. Several studies also show a link to sleep too long and an increased risk of stroke. However, it is likely that it is a marker and no cause for stroke, the researcher adds. Some people get by in a shorter time; others need a little more than average, but crossing the border of sleep habits seems to be a bad omen.

ENVIRONMENTAL CHANGES

Over the past few decades, more and more people are having lower sleep quality; we do not get enough qualitative sleep. The biggest problem seems to be a lack of ability to relax at the end of the day. The highest priority is to find something quick and easy to use when sleep does not come naturally.

Our society spins faster and faster each year and soon we are half artificial. The prediction of human achievement in the near future says that by 2050, the human brain has lost to computer. At that time, the computer matches the human brain in all respects. But we are not there yet. We are still 100% humans with all our weaknesses and strengths.

At the beginning of my sleep studies, I came across figures that reflect our past and our future. Numbers are interesting to look at, knowing that some may not be completely accurate. However, the figures give an immediate experience and everyone knows that these parameters have changed tremendously over the past two centuries.

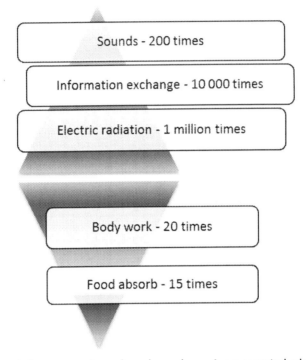

Figure 1 Increased and reduced environmental changes

The industrial revolution, with extensive social, economic and technological advances, began in the late 18th century and began the industrialization of the world. The industrial revolution became increasingly important when steam-powered vessels and railways became increasingly common.

During the 19th century the transformation spread to the rest of Western Europe, North America and Japan, later to the rest of the world. The consequence was extensive movements of population, from rural to urban industrial communities, and the pace of everything measurably increased each year.

The second industrial revolution is usually referred to the time of the late 1800s and to the First World War. The spread of electrical engineering and the use of electricity marked this time, but also of the combustion engine and steel production. The genius Tesla was involved in this period and he invented the AC technique, how to displace electric current over long distances.

It would not be difficult to propagate personal computers, the mobile phone and the World Wide Web as the third industrial revolution of modern times. Before the World Wide Web was invented, there were no systems to easily link to and the WWW came from a project at the European research center CERN, the world's largest particle physics laboratory and in the early 90s the rights were released free.

ELECTRIC RADIATION

With this historical background, it is no wonder humans get hard to keep up, increasingly connected and electric radiation surrounds us all the time. In a recent Finnish study, the mobile phone has an impact on childbirth, and fewer children are born in Finland. This study focuses on the mobile's psychologically dependent factors. The researchers argue that the mobile phone affects couples relationships; one is not interested enough for a socializing and eventually becomes too tired.

More and more people are exposed to electromagnetic fields from electrical appliances, power lines, mobile telephony and other wireless communications. This gives rise to concerns and concerns that the increased exposure could affect health negatively. There are established biological facts from acute exposure at high levels explained by recognized biophysical mechanisms. External ELF magnetic fields induce electric fields and currents in the body which, at very high field strengths, cause nerve and muscle stimulation and changes in the nerve cell's legibility in the central nervous system. The latest global increase in the use of wireless communication has resulted in greater exposure to radio frequency electromagnetic fields (RF-EMF). The brain is the main target of the radiation when the phones are used, with the highest exposure on the same side of the brain where the phone is located. Children and adolescents are more exposed to radiation than adults because of their thinner skull and smaller head. The brain is still developing up to 20 years of age and up to that time it is relatively vulnerable. Much of the scientific research that researches long-term risks from ELF magnetic field exposure has focused on child leukemia. Analyzes of epidemiological studies show a consistent pattern of a two-fold increase in childhood leukemia, associated with average frequency magnetic field exposure. Researchers have conducted an overall analysis of two case control studies on malignant brain tumors in patients aged 18-80 years. Only cases with histopathological control of the tumor were included. Mobile phone use increased the risk of glioma by 95%. The highest risk found for glioma was in the temporal lobe. The first use of mobile or wireless telephone before the age of 20 gave higher results for glioma than in later age groups.

Mobile research does not agree whether there is a risk. An Interphone study 2011 failed to find strong evidence for increased risk, yet a large Prospective study 2013 on cancer and radiation between middle-aged British women. The study, however, had serious methodological problems according to controlling researchers. Electric radiation surrounds us all the time and the new construction of G-technology is gaining more space in our lives. There was a higher risk for third generation (3G) mobile phone use compared to other types (GSM), but this was based on short latency and fairly low number of exposed participants, the authors say. 3G telecommunications systems mobile phones provide broadband microwave signals, which "hypothetically" can result in higher biological effects compared to other signals, the researchers concluded.

The idea is not new; the physicist Tesla had great plans for passing electricity through the air. The technology was so long before its time, that it didn't become real. Today's technology will benefit many people in their daily lives and provide a link to, above all, sparsely populated areas, services that provide both jobs and service. The welfare will reach out to everyone, is the common message. However, this is not always beneficial as the electrification exposes our bodies to radiation that is not normal. Electricity sensitivity is a medical concept, but an opposite relationship to the whole planning of modern society. But if one has known of the symptoms, then it is very real and the whole organism is knocked out. Human cells work by means of electrical stimulation through the sodium / calcium pump. The protein pump in the cell membrane contributes to sodium having a higher concentration outside the cell than inside and calcium reversed.

An electric machine that knocks out is short-circuited by too much electricity, grounded according to all technical capabilities. A machine seems to have a value that must be preserved. The human body also cannot resist too much electricity. One might think that this subject is overlooked by the rulers, but will be a major problem in the future. This problem might be worse, than the problems in our external environment, such as water and air pollution in shorter perspective.

The Swedish Radiation Safety Authority believes that today there is no scientific support for the fact that mobile radiation is actually harmful, but for reasons of caution people at the same time has to reduce exposure. The authority usually refers to the fact that one cannot see any overall threat or damage picture in general for humanity. But this may change according to recent rapports; the male fertility has halved in 50 years. It can be that bad; in a hundred years is only every fifth man or fewer, capable of producing children. For some reason, the man's ability in this regard has radically deteriorated. This goes hand in hand with a galloping increase in insomnia that spreads around our planet. There are probably several different reasons for this scenario, such as several dangerous chemicals in nature. But it can also be an overly expanded grid, as well as mobiles and computers that make the cells' work performance worse. Now that 4G is also expanded, the successor 5G is also planned.

Many researchers agree that this may involve radiation doses that can result in incurable injuries. The transfer rate will require denser mobile base stations at every 10 houses in an ordinary residential area. In their letter, doctors and scientists write: "We recommend a moratorium on the expansion of the fifth generation of telecommunications, until potential risks to human health and the environment have been fully investigated by industry-independent researchers."The appeal has now been signed by 230 researchers from 41 nations - all have published scientific articles on the effects of electromagnetic fields.

In any case, it does not harm to do a thorough independent scientific study on how radiation affects humans in the short and long term. A Risk Day exercise came in 2010 on Electricity Sensitivity; Motion 2010/11: F249, which gives hope for draft decisions. Justification: Electricity sensitivity is about to become a major public health problem, especially for those who are affected but also for society as a whole. According to the National Board of Health and Welfare's calculations, more than 280,000 people are present in our country, and about one-tenth of these have serious problems. One might wonder what happened in eight years, after the motion became public. The future may provide answers.

BODY WORK

With the help of the computer society, we become increasingly seated in front of screens. Especially children and adolescents move less and less in a few decades ago. The body uses a certain amount of energy during the day without physical activity, when the individual is awake but is at rest. Generally, one usually expects 34kkal per kilogram of body weight, which also varies with age. It may seem that basal metabolism requires so much that one should be able to eat what one wants but without exercising, but reality shows another way. Basal metabolism is the energy consumption at rest required for the organs to function, which is affected by body size, physical activity, age and sex. Basal metabolism varies from person to person and is partly controlled by the genome. What influences is, among other things, how good the body is in absorbing food, storing and burning it. Basal metabolism is generally higher for men than for women.

The various components of the energy conversion, in a moderately active person who moves at least 30 minutes / day on a moderate to high intensity, correspond to: Basal metabolism 60%, Food metabolism 10%, Everyday movements and physical exercise 30%. Too sedentary life, especially in the early age, constitutes a negative spiral for society as a whole. Man works best with some form of regular movement for the cells to function and not be damaged. Too many cell injuries may cause dysfunction and disease.

SUMMARY

Environmental change in society seems to increase year by year. The faster communication between people makes it more difficult with own time, always connected.

***

Research shows that microwave radiation from computers, mobile phones and WiFi causes cancer, damages the reproductive capacity, the brain and the function of the central nervous system.

***

Never use cell phones directly against the head. Mobile with the speaker function or a hands-free is preferred.

***

Turn off broadband routers in the home when not in use.

***

Research shows that electromagnetic radiation interferes with sleep.

***

Less movement makes the human body more susceptible to stress.

Stress

Stress is something we all have to deal with to varying degrees. Some have a high stress threshold; others suffer long periods of abnormal stress levels. If you feel stressed in life and have problems with chronic fatigue, depression and memory impairment, it may be signs of adrenal fatigue. Stress is an antagonist of normal sleep behavior. Stress can be handled well if you get enough sleep, but when sleep starts to deteriorate too much you are in trouble and the term "hit the wall" is used.

In recent years, it has become increasingly recognized that worry and stress are very prominent in the adult population. The frequency is about twice as many among women. Studies have shown that anxiety causes morbidity, utilization of health care services, disability. Relaxation training is increasingly common form of treatment for concern. Many studies support relaxation training to reduce anxiety, and stress

Here, the therapeutic use of relaxation techniques can be considered particularly relevant, the observable effects clear and, moreover, as part of healthier lifestyle changes. The researchers nevertheless agree that further studies are necessary to elucidate the complex physiology behind the relaxation response and its impact on stress-related disease states.

Exposure to chronic stress prevented normal weight gain in both male and female rats. The rats were under intense stress twice daily for fifteen days. Researchers also found that levels of stress hormone corticosterone, adrenal cortical steroid, were much higher in female rats exposed to chronic stress than in male rats. The steroid is released by the adrenal glands in response to stress in the same pattern as the stress hormone cortisol is released in humans.

There are various ways to look at stress. Less stress can

be defined as acute stress over a few hours. High stress levels can be over days or weeks. Cumulative stress, successively adding stress can be just as important as or more important than individual specific stressors. This means the increasing effects of daily doses of what we eat, drinks, smoking habits, work, sleep quality and so on. Lifetime exposure of stress is believed to exert its influence through a "risk chain", where early exposure to adverse events increases the risk of later exposures in an ongoing negative feedback loop. It affects physical, mental and behavioral outcomes such as the occurrence of high blood pressure, physical disability, pain and other chronic diseases. Physiological pathways that link cumulative stress to physical illness have not yet been fully understood, according to researchers.

Both cumulative stress and insufficient exercise are associated with poorer health. Stress is related to muscle / skeletal problems and a decrease in physical function over time. There are several sources of evidence to support the perception of an interaction between stress and exercise. For example, among older adults, physical health symptoms are greatest in those with both little training and high perceived stress. Those who do not exercise have a higher incidence of type II diabetes and coronary artery disease, including health outcomes. In addition, interventions aimed at increasing exercise have resulted in reductions in physical diseases, such as high blood pressure. Women also tend to report more symptoms of stress and new research suggests that women are less protected by training from stress-related ailments. The combination of strenuous exercise and high stress levels can result in a health-hazardous state of physiological overload - too much is bad and yet too little.

Exercise is associated with subdued sympathetic and cardiovascular stress reactivity when exposed to stressful stimuli. A controlled study showed that both exercise and stress management significantly improved the flow and expansion of the brachial artery. There seems to be a minimum physical activity level needed to achieve such effects: 150 minutes of moderate-to-severe physical activity per week has been shown to optimize physical health, according to some researchers.

Acute stress for a short time has all experienced, in school, jobs and relationships, but when this develops into long chronic periods, this means a serious tension for the whole body. All systems become affected and sleep usually becomes the first important loss and everything becomes a vicious spiral. In some results, mental stress showed a decrease of almost 30 percent of the blood flow to the brain. In addition, doctors are increasingly talking about the severity of stress and its impact on the heart. According to the researcher; Stress-induced reduction in blood flow to the heart is more common than previously thought. Several studies indicated psychological stresses were among the most important risk factors for death in heart patients. One study showed that for some patients, mental stress is as dangerous as smoking cigarettes or having high cholesterol. Scientists are not sure if chronically stressed people are less likely to have healthy lifestyles, or if people with unhealthy habits tend to feel more stressed at work. To be aware of your own stress, you should consider your lifestyle and above all make sure your sleep is of reasonably good quality.

Everyone knows that stress normally has a negative impact on sleep. I wrote "normally" because there is such a factor as "positive stress". Positive stress, or flow, means a state of mind when you act according to your purpose and aim both physically and mentally. You do something you can handle and like. With positive stress, time flies and you do not have control over the time scale, the time dimension seems to disappear. You work in a vacuum. All your senses focus only on one thing, you work in a flow that you have control over. This period of positive stress has no negative effect. Normally you fall asleep with a smile. Think or dream about next day's escapades, even if you have worked more than normal number of working hours. It seems that having control and doing something that is interesting is of great importance to the physical health.

The adrenal glands are the glands that primarily respond

to our stress response, both long-term and short-lived. In stress, the nervous system sends signals to the adrenal glands, which in turn release hormones into the blood. These hormones are adrenaline and norepinephrine, both of which account for the first activation in your stress response and later also cortisol, which accounts for the sustained stress response.

When our adrenal glands have been over activated for too long, they can end up in such a high degree of fatigue that the ability to respond to stress is greatly weakened and the recovery is made difficult. Adrenal insufficiency is when the adrenal gland releases too little of the hormone cortisol and sometimes aldosterone. Symptoms usually include fatigue, upset stomach, dehydration, and skin changes. Signs of physical and mental symptoms of fatigue are for at least two weeks. The most prominent is clear lack of energy. This may be manifested in reduced endurance or prolonged recovery time associated with mental stress. Important hormones:

Adrenaline works partly as cortisol, but is much stronger and seems more short-term. The extra adrenaline causes symptoms like rapid heart rhythm, palpitations, tremors, weaknesses and mood swings.

Aldosterone is part of the body's salt and water balance and affects blood pressure.

Cortisol is an anti-inflammatory hormone; stabilize the blood sugar, stimulate the immune system and maintain the muscle mass. The cortisol levels are highest in the morning.

During chronic stress for a long time, the adrenal glands will not be able to produce the amount of cortisol you need without affecting other hormones. Over time, sleep problems develop and even if sleep has occurred, you do not feel rested. Over time, adrenal glands become exhausted and cortisol levels begin to decline. The body goes into energy-saving mode to survive and begins to break down muscle tissue to produce energy, which causes you to lose muscle tissue and no longer manage to exercise.

Abbreviated telomere length, the end portion of the

chromosomes, is known to be associated with aging, but also associated with depression and hypocortisolism. Findings confirm previous research showing shorter telomer length in depressed patients. HPA (Hypothalamic-Pituitary-Adrenal) which is a very important regulator of stress response, best known for cortisol regulation. Normally, stress shows an increased incidence of the hormone cortisol, but new studies show that chronic stress instead turns off the cortisol, so-called hypokortisol. The condition is associated with high C-reactive protein, inflammation levels. Hypochlorisolism has been found in patients with:

- Chronic fatigue syndrome
- Post-traumatic stress disorder
- Burnout
- Fibromyalgia
- Irritable bowel syndrome

Disorders that share symptoms of fatigue, pain and increased stress sensitivity. Traditionally, too much cortisol has been considered harmful, but the opposite is also true, according to researchers. When you experience chronic stress, a too high stress level over time, cortisol levels go down. In chronic stress, HPA cannot deliver cortisol, but turns off the cortisol.

SUMMARY

Cortisol is an anti-inflammatory hormone; stabilize the blood sugar, stimulate the immune system and maintain the muscle mass. The cortisol levels are highest in the morning.

***

Relaxation training is increasingly common treatment for concern. Many studies support relaxation exercise to reduce anxiety, anxiety and stress.

***

At higher levels of increasing stress, sometimes training fails to provide health benefits, but instead gives a premium of higher stress levels and blood pressure. On these occasions, relaxation periods are preferred, before regular exercise begins.

***

During stress, the cortisol increases to protect, but with chronic stress over time, cortisol levels go down. HPA does not deliver cortisol, but turns off, hypocortisol. The term "enter the wall" is then used.

***

Cortisol, the hypothesis for promoting fear, HPG and testosterone, promotes reward seeking, HPA, in Amygdala.

***

Insomnia

Having a good night's sleep and, above all, enough deep sleep is probably the most important parameter for a long and healthy life. William Dement, professor of psychiatry at Stanford University, found a link between sleep and health. He said: "To maintain good health, sleep can be more critical than diet, exercise and even heredity."

A meeting and reflection to describe the headline's medical facts - I talked to a stranger and we soon began to discuss sleep-related problems. Sleep you can be without, at least three or four days, he said. His record went to five nights without any sleep at all. His secret was to keep his focus and he was very determined by his statement. How much immune deficiency do you get from five nights of sleep? At the end of our discussion, he still said it was the truth and nothing but the truth. Then I thought he was completely wrong out there, but after a bit of research I have to give him partly right. Considering how one reacted after just one night of poor sleep, it is still difficult to understand and react with five nights without any sleep at all.

The record of alertness is more than double, more than eleven nights. But it was under scientific control and not loneliness escaped. The record was made in the 70s by American Randy Gardner. Gardner often had data to solve, to test motor skills and memory ability. Already on the second day, Gardner had problems focusing his vision and during his third day there was a strong mood swing. It must be much harder to keep focus as a single, lonely person. There is no one to help you stay awake, even if you are determined and focused person. However, it is relatively common to have the wrong opinion or facts about your own sleep skills. Sometimes the feeling of being awake all night is rarely right. People often sleep at times, even if the important deep sleep first fails, instead periods of REM sleep can occur.

A Swedish study found that a poor psychosocial work environment led to a more than twice the risk of developing a new episode of insomnia compared to normal sleeping. Insomnia shows increased metabolism, as body temperature and heart rate. Insomnia patients also exhibit higher levels of cortisol, suggesting increased activity in the stress response system. These data suggest that individuals show consistent sleep responses to stressors and those individuals with higher sympathetic activation may be more susceptible to developing insomnia. The results showed that it may be possible to detect vulnerability to insomnia and that such vulnerability is associated with hyperarousal. Arousal levels at bedtime show the relationship between stresses during the day and sleep disturbances the following night. When mental stress raises blood pressure it can be a risk factor for high blood pressure. Meanwhile, blood pressure rises with mental stress, but the change varies in level from person to person. "If a person experiences more than a 20 percent increase in blood pressure due to mental stress, it is an abnormal activation of the sympathetic nervous system that can damage blood vessels and vital organs," researchers say. Mental stress can thus be associated with organ damage.

Sleep should be considered as an important part of the workplace's health, researchers call for a new study. Workers who experience insomnia and other sleep-related problems are less productive during the working day, losing twice as much productivity. Those who reported only 5 to 6 hours of sleep reported 19% more productivity loss and those who received less than 5 hours of sleep showed 50% more productivity loss. In the hope of being more productive, the sleep time goes down, but in the long run this strategy does not work. Sleep is not a time expense but an investment, the researchers concluded.

Sleep disturbance causes negative health effects and poor quality of life. People with sleep disorders have higher levels of depression and anxiety and increased cardiovascular disease. Women have a higher incidence than men of insomnia and depression, associated with poor sleep and are more likely than men to complain of insomnia, headache, irritability and fatigue. The type of complaint differs significantly between the sexes, according to researchers.

The results of a study indicate that the factors that cause insomnia are different for young people of different ages. Genetic factors, varying with age, contribute to insomnia in children and teenagers. The estimated incidence of insomnia varies between 4% and 41% in early childhood and adolescence. The researchers were most surprised that the genetic factors were not stable over time, so the influence of genes also depends on the child's development.

Insomnia is a condition seen throughout the world. In a random phone survey in the United States, about 33% of adult sleep disorders reported, who performed regularly in 9% of respondents. One third of adults reports that it is difficult to fall asleep in the last 12 months, and 17 percent report this problem as a significant one. Insomnia can be acute or chronic. In a recent Swedish study, it was found that almost 50 percent of the Swedish population needed to improve their sleep, which then had increased from just over 30 percent. Insomnia is an extremely common condition with major social and economic consequences worldwide. Insomnia is a diffuse disease with significant socio-economic consequences and often presents with a number of associated pathologies that affect the condition of the prognosis. In case of insufficient treatment, insomnia may become chronic and increasingly severe.

Mental disorders are often associated with insomnia. An epidemiological study reported that individuals with insomnia have a 4.5-fold higher probability of presenting depression compared to those with normal sleep patterns. In addition, patients with insomnia have an increased risk of showing depression within 3.5 years of onset, even in the absence of mental disorders. In short, people with sleep disorder have higher susceptibility to depression and people with depression are more likely to achieve insomnia than healthy individuals.

Chronic insomnia also has many health effects and is associated with higher health care, including a 2-fold increase in hospital stays, such as depression, anxiety, alcohol dependence, drug addiction, and suicide.

Chronic sleep deprivation, fragmented sleep results in excessive sleepiness, neurocognitive dysfunction, memory loss, deprezion and worst case cause heart rhythm abnormalities. Sleep restriction is also associated with a 28% increase in the daytime level of the hormone ghrelin, which contributes to increased appetite and weight gain among patients with insomnia.

GREHLIN

In one study, cognitive abilities, memory and motor skills were measured after sleep deprivation and found that those who regularly missed sleep became more or less toxic, which also been shown by animal experiments. After just four hours of sleep, the body has difficulty regulating blood sugar, which compensates for energy loss by releasing hormones to compensate for the lack of energy-reducing leptin in blood plasma and increasing the amount of ghrelin. This compensation creates a strong demand for heavier carbohydrates. Sleeping too little causes you to eat more and it can cause obesity for some people. If you eat over the limit of carbohydrates you risk stabilizing a high level of insulin, and this may end up in a life-threatening future scenario of negative conditions. Ghrelin has an important influence on the nerves, especially in the hippocampus, and is essential for cognitive adaptation and learning process.

Another study: Among other hormonal effects, researchers found that sleep restriction caused an increase in ghrelin levels in the blood. Ghrelin is a hormone that has been shown to reduce energy, stimulate hunger and food intake, promote fat deposits and increase glucose production in the body. This may explain why sleep deprived participants also reported feeling hunger during the study. Ghrelin is mainly excreted from the stomach and stimulates appetite and growth hormone (GH) release. Studies have shown that ghrelin has a wide range of functions. In the gastrointestinal tract, ghrelin affects several functions, including gastric acid secretion.

Sleeping less means you eat more and increase in weight. For some people this can mean obesity. Glucose-PET studies have shown that after twenty-four hours of long-term alertness, sleep deprivation results primarily in the decrease of immune function and growth hormones. Sleep is one of the events that change the timing of secretion for some hormones. Many hormones are secreted into the blood during sleep. Researchers believe that the release of growth hormone is related to repair processes that occur during sleep.

SUMMARY

*T*o maintain good health, sleep can be more critical than diet, exercise and even heredity.

***

*I*nsomnia shows increased metabolic rate, body temperature and heart rate.

***

*I*nsomnia patients also exhibit higher levels of cortisol, suggesting increased activity in the stress response system

***

*P*eople with sleep disorder have higher susceptibility to depression and people with depression are more likely to achieve insomnia than healthy individuals.

***

*C*hronic insomnia associated with impaired occupational and social performance and an elevated absence of 10 times greater than control groups.

***

*I*nsomnia appears to be predictive of a number of disorders, including depression, anxiety, alcohol dependence, drug addiction and suicide.

***

*S*leep restriction caused an increase in the ghrelin level in the blood. Ghrelin is a hormone that has been shown to reduce energy, stimulate hunger and food intake, promote fat retention and increase glucose production in the body.

***

*A*fter twenty-four hours of long-term alertness, sleep deprivation results primarily in the decrease of immune function and growth hormones.

***

*C*hanging the nervous system for the night is a key function and entering the alpha rhythm promotes the entrance to sleep.

***

Circadian rhythm

Good sleep brings with it many parameters and systems that must work in unison. Small deviation sometimes causes imbalance of myriads of molecules. A weak sleep engine must be compensated, nothing comes naturally. A process that controls sleep is a circadian rhythm, which is built-in and regularly cyclical with a period of about one day, in living organisms. Such rhythms exist in a large number of organisms, plants and animals. The human body has adapted to daily changes of light and darkness, so it anticipates periods of sleep and activity. Deviations from this circadian rhythm come with functional consequences. The inner biological clocks control a number of other processes, such as metabolism, food intake and changes between rest and activity.

Everyone, even those with good sleep, certainly have many examples of events where the circadian rhythm played a punch. For example; when one suddenly wakes up the clear wake seemingly for no reason at all. It is when this happens often, more often than exception, as it becomes a permanent problem. Perhaps several time a week and even if you keep a strict sleep diary, it can be difficult to isolate a particular cause. It is probably the body rhythm that runs freely and sleep is switched to alertness.

People are different, exhibit individual differences in circadian rhythm and can be divided into morning or night people or neither. This is very much due to our genetic background. Since the diurnal bell is slightly longer than 24 hours and also varies in length from person to person, the daily rhythm therefore tends to shift to varying degrees. A strong sleep engine can withstand a variation in the circadian rhythm, but a poorly-drawn person cannot resist a dysfunction in the rhythm.

The homeostatic process represents the balance between sleep and alertness, so that insufficient sleep leads to increased sleepiness. The system promotes sleep and alertness in a ratio of about 1 to 2, giving about 8 hours of sleep over a 24-hour period. When a person is awake from morning to bedtime, there is a steady build up of homeostatic sleepiness that is picked out when the night begins. While the hemostatic process determines the desired amount of sleep, the circadian process optimizes sleep to occur during the night. Sleep is facilitated by high homeostatic levels during the early part of the night, but the homeostatic level decays during the night. Sleep can normally continue during the latter part of the night due to minimal circadian stimulation, which effectively promotes sleepiness, up to normal awakening.

People who have worked night shifts fall asleep the following morning due to the onset of homeostatic sleepiness, but often it can be difficult to get sleep stable due to the time of the circadian rhythm. The alertness is promoted by many neurotransmitters such as glutamate, acetylcholine, dopamine, serotonin and histamine. Exactly what happens during alertness is not completely clear.

MOLECULAR CLOCK AND SKELETAL MUSCLE

The fact that muscles are an important attribute of the circadian rhythm is becoming increasingly apparent, as more facts and research are presented at an ever-faster rate. The story behind the clock genes is young and the first article defining circadian genes in skeletal muscle was published in 2007 and identified 215, but up-dated research extended the list to more than 2,300 genes. The importance of the muscles status of human well-being rises after which more genes are found in the future.

The molecular watch is present in virtually all cells and the skeletal muscle is one of the largest organs, almost half of the total body mass. Clock genes participate in a wide range of functions, including muscle development and metabolism. When circadian rhythms are disturbed, the observed effect on skeletal muscle is:

- Change of fiber type in muscles
- Mitochondrial and muscle dysfunction

Side effects of metabolic seakness include impaired glucose tolerance and insulin sensitivity. It is well known that the skeletal muscles work to produce power and motion, reserves of amino acids and also as a depot for glucose. Overlapping research has been especially noted in association studies of metabolic markers and disease. Thus, risk variants from genes traditionally related to sleep regulation have been shown to be associated with obesity and type 2 diabetes markers. Thus, genetic data points to a number of pathways that link sleep, circadian rhythm, metabolism, and disease. This clearly shows that exercise and exercise are even more important for our health and sleep than previously thought.

Changes in muscle composition and function are also strongly correlated with disease development. Two of the most common diseases, cardiovascular disease and cancer are associated with loss of muscle mass, decreased strength and impaired muscle metabolism. In particular, severe loss of muscle mass is a significant risk factor for mortality in these disease states. Another common health problem, diabetes, is linked to skeletal muscle function, where reduced insulin sensitivity in the skeletal muscle is involved in the onset of type 2 diabetes.

The SCN molecule clock communicates with other tissues, e.g. as the skeletal muscle. The skeletal muscle molecule clock is governed by factors such as light, time for meals and activity. It is in this indirect way that the skeletal muscle clock is modulated by light rays. Circadic rhythm is driven by the molecular clock, which in mammals sometimes involves other core clock genes: Bmal1 and Clock.

BMA1 AND CLOCK

The circadian clock network is an evolutionarily conserved mechanism that regulates various biological processes. BMAL1 (Brain-Muscle-Arnt-Like 1) is an essential transcriptional activator at DNA level and is strongly expressed in the skeletal muscle. Muscle-specific loss of BMAL1 resulted in decreased uptake of skeletal muscle glucose, decreased glucose oxidation. Studies suggest that muscle-specific conservation of BMA1 may be sufficient to increase longevity. Many common diseases are associated with altered muscle mass, function and metabolism, as well as cancer and heart disease. These diseases are linked to changes in the skeletal muscles. The molecular clock, as in the BMA1 gene, significantly affects metabolism in skeletal muscles.

Almost all spinal cells have self-contained clocks that pair endogenous rhythms with changes in the cell environment. Genetic disorder of clock genes in mice causes disrupted metabolic function of specific tissues at distinct stages of sleep / waking cycle. Lack of BMAL1 in mice has impaired circadian behavior. Studies have shown that reduced BMAL1 in mice has reduced lifespans and shows various symptoms of premature aging including sarcoplasia, cataracts, minor subcutaneous fat and organ shrinkage.

Lack of CLOCK protein significantly affects longevity. The average CLOCK in mice is reduced by 15% compared to wild mice, while the maximum lifetime is reduced by more than 20%. The result suggests that CLOCK plays an important role in aging and is crucial for regulating normal physiology. Their free running period of about 24 hours is temperature compensated. This means that biological clocks do not go slower at lower temperatures or increase when it gets warmer. Study indicates that the circadian clock in skeletal muscle is sensitive to scheduled exercise in a normal light environment. In addition, the researchers found; 4 weeks of low intensity endurance training is sufficient to substantially correct the clock.

In banana flies, a biological clock rhythm has been found

in many different cells, some of which react directly to light. In higher vertebrates, the CLOCK function is in the eyes, the pine gland and the SCN. The fact that one can influence people's circadian rhythm by illuminating the knee folds provides further nourishment to a number of questions about the function of our inner clock and how it is regulated. If there are several different biological clocks, they must, for example, communicate with each other.

SUMMARY

Biological clocks control a number of processes, such as metabolic, food intake and changes between rest and activity.

∗∗∗

While the hemostatic process determines the desired amount of sleep, the circadian process optimizes sleep to occur during the night.

∗∗∗

People who have worked with night shifts fall asleep the following morning due to the onset of homeostatic sleepiness, but often have difficulty getting sleep stable due to the time of the circadian system.

∗∗∗

Genetic disorder of clock genes in mice causes disturbed metabolic function of specific tissues at distinct stages of sleep / waking cycle.

∗∗∗

Studies suggest that muscle-specific conservation of Bmal1 may be sufficient to increase longevity.

∗∗∗

Study indicates that the circadian clock in skeletal muscle is sensitive to scheduled exercise in a normal light environment.

∗∗∗

When circadian rhythms are disturbed, the observed effect on skeletal muscle is: fiber-type shifts, mitochondrial and muscle dysfunction

∗∗∗

Muscles and
sleep in space

To address this issue, muscles and sleep to an extreme level, think of "sleep in space". How can astronauts in space have anything to do with ordinary earthly people and their environment, what is the connection?

Sixty plus years of space research is a short period in human development, but if you are sufficiently old, there are many memories of rocket launches from the early 70s. Jury Gagarin, the first man in orbit around the world (April 1961) and who started the race against the United States, in Vostok 1. John Glenn then copied the space flight from Cape Canaveral, but reinforced the historic moment with three laps around the Earth in Friendskip 7 (Feb 1962).

We all know how we sleep on the surface of the earth. It is an environment that we understand and have references to. How about sleeping in orbit around the earth? It is not common to sit in a spaceship on weekends, but now private investors want to get their share of the space cake and make preparations to get gravity-free travel. Astronauts and cosmonauts, with several names, have the special expertise for space missions. But air travel without gravity, are there differences in sleep length and quality?

We have seen through the television, how crew members live and work during their space visits. From history, we know that astronauts from different countries have reached stationary orbits and are weightless, Zero-G. This special effect makes a difference when working and living in space, the stabilization from gravity is not there. One has to think about how to perform in other ways, such as daily earthly tasks; to eat, go to the toilet, sleep. But sleep is a separate chapter, you are weightless and floating around, you get into stationary sleeping bags that are sealed. But all this knows most and has seen. But the question is, what sleep quality can be expected in a weightless orbit around the earth? Are there any differences between Earth-G and Zero-G? Is it harder to fall asleep in the orbit around the earth? The 24-hour day and night rhythm (circadian rhythm) is disturbed, as the craft in the track counts in minutes, not hours. Can sleep be maintained, get enough sleep, compared to Earth? An interesting question: Is it allowed for astronauts to take sleep medicine if they can't sleep? Can we learn something about sleeping in space, which we can use back on the ground?

If you do some exploration of - sleep in space, you will find that crew members may have difficulty sleeping during space flight. Despite its advanced training for several years, is it different to circulate in circulation for the first time? New impressions usually have a bad effect on sleep, especially for ordinary people. A combination of factors contributes to their sleep problems:

- Exitment
- Closed environment
- High quality tasks
- Absence of normal day / night cycles

Although NASA's recommendations provide for astronauts to sleep for 8 hours, it is not commonplace. Studies show that astronauts normally sleep 0.5 to 2.5 hours less than they do on Earth. Many astronauts report that they feel completely restored after just six hours of sleep. Can less gravity have something to do with better rest periods for some astronaut in an orbit? But I assume the same share of space as on earth; some have good sleep, others do not.

How about 10% of industrial worlds regularly use sleep pills? What can be presumed by a skilled trained astronaut? Well, to improve sleep, many astronauts take sleep aids such as benzodiazepine, according to research documents. Many astronauts have to take pills to sleep. In fact, sleep pills account for almost half of the entire arsenal of drugs used in space. But spacecraft doesn't get as much sleep as they usually get on earth. Not getting enough sleep hours can affect their duties. Although they do not have enough sleep, they normally have to perform the daily routine. However, the use of sleep medication has an effect the following day, due to unwanted side effects on performance and mental attention.

At the beginning of the Gemini flights, some planned maneuvers must be interrupted due to astronate fatigue. For most Skylab flights (flights 3 and 4), biomedical changes were seen, such as decreased cardiac activity and decreased skeletal muscle strength. Generally, the conclusion was drawn, changed work routines showed better performance with 4 hours of work after 4 hours of rest, so-called 4: 4 schedule.

A factor related to circadian rhythm applies to the variables that regulate the 24-hour clock. Such variables are called zeitgebers; a wide range of physical, temporal and social signals that serve to bring sleep and alertness to a particular rhythm. A specialist report concluded that the time has little significance in space flights, in addition to performing work routines and personal communication. When zeitgebers are not present, some rhythms become "free" and thus may vary from a 24-hour schedule. The assumption that artificial lighting will function as a major contributing factor to periodicity, but some studies indicate that social signals may be even more important than light conditions for regulating work performance. Early shuttle flights showed that the crew often slept poorly in space due to old technology and small spacecraft, etc. The 90-minute orbit meant that the astronauts have daylight and darkness changes every 45 minutes, which after a while destroys their body clock.

A basic question, if "normal" sleep patterns can ever be achieved in space? During later Apollo missions, the amount and quality of sleep was still unresolved. For example, astronauts reported difficulty finding a place to rest their head, discomfort in the astronaut suit, all combined contributing to inferior sleep. The sleep conditions improved during the Skylab mission and some encouraging results were reported. The length of sleep, or the time needed to fall asleep, was relatively long in the early parts of the 84-day mission. In the later half of the mission the sleep conditions returned to values typical of pre and post flight conditions. No significant change in sleep pattern is seen in 59-day assignments. Surprisingly, the most marked changes in sleep occurred during adaptation to a 1-G, which could be more disturbing to sleep than adaptation to a 0-G.

Skeletal muscle atrophy is evident after lack of muscle work during space flights. The study shows that the atrophic processes are rapidly and within 72 hours of lack of muscle work and suggests that countermeasures should be used in the early stages of space missions to compensate or prevent muscle loss during the period of muscle atrophy.

Skeletal muscle atrophy is evident after lack of muscle work during space flights. The study shows that the atrophic processes are rapidly and within 72 hours of lack of muscle work and suggests that countermeasures should be used in the early stages of space missions to compensate or prevent muscle loss during the period of muscle atrophy.

Interesting for future studies; good sleep is better achieved in space and not dependent on muscle status, comparing with the Earth's 1 g environment. One of the most important issues for this book is to explain that sleep status may be dependent on muscle types. The fact that astronauts have more sleep problems returned to Earth would support the theory that 1G - high muscle dependence and 0G - muscle independence.

Is it a fact; sleep in space is better? Studies have shown that micro gravity has a deep negative response within a wide range of physiological parameters. Strength training has positively affected key markers of muscle atrophy. NASA develops and tests new and innovative technologies that enable the future of safe and effective human exploration. Exercise training (resistance + aerobic exercise) on the M-MED (Multi-Mode Exercise

Device) device has positively affected muscle function and improves aerobic capacity. This device is designed to maintain the astronauts' cardiovascular system, muscle and skeletal characteristics by providing muscle strength and endurance training with low resistance. Researchers address the problem of muscle loss in space and hope to find solutions that will also benefit people with muscle weakening on Earth.

In a weightless environment, astronauts quickly lose muscle mass. On the ground, similar muscle loss occurs in the elderly and people who are confined to their beds. Growth hormone in combination with strength training is crucial for maintaining muscle strength.

Despite NASA recommendations that astronauts should sleep 8 hours a day in space, sleep is usually limited in spaceflight, averaging 0.5 hours to 2.5 hours during astronauts' basic sleep times, NASA researchers say. Six studies over 25 years of age have documented average daily sleep time in space flying between 4.0 and 6.5 hours and acute total sleep loss (24-36 hours without sleep) may also occur before critical surgery.

Life on Earth has evolved to coincide with daylight and darkness, which derive from our planet's 24-hour rotation. Like other animals, man has an internal biological clock that acts as a biological watchman. The watch prepares the body and the mind for restful sleep at night and active alertness during the day.

An experiment consisting of three sleep applications was designed to study the effects of space flight on crew members before, during and after spaceflight. Changes in rapid eye movement (REM) sleep with adaptation to microgravity and rewriting to a 1-G environment were studied. Preliminary analyzes showed that REM sleep was greatly reduced during the flight for all five astronauts. Both REM time and REM% (of total sleep time) decreased significantly. On average, REM time was greatly reduced during flight compared to preflight. There was also a reduction in total sleep time during the flight. All persons showed reductions in average nightly total sleep time. This was not due to a reduction in bed time; they spent an average of 4% longer in bed during flight. Rather, it was due to reduced sleep efficiency.

An experiment consisting of three sleep applications was designed to study the effects of space flight on crew members before, during and after spaceflight. Changes in rapid eye movement (REM) sleep with adaptation to microgravity and rewriting to a 1-G environment were studied. Preliminary analyzes showed that REM sleep was greatly reduced during the flight for all five astronauts. Both REM time and REM% (of total sleep time) decreased significantly. On average, REM time was greatly reduced during flight compared to preflight. There was also a reduction in total sleep time during the flight. All persons showed reductions in average nightly total sleep time. This was not due to a reduction in bedtime; they spent an average of 4% longer in bed during flight. Rather, it was due to reduced sleep efficiency.

The astronauts lose 10 to 20 percent of their muscle mass on short missions. On long-term flights, such as the Russian space station MIR or the International Space Station, muscle loss can rise to 50 percent without using countermeasures. A clear change in the depletion of muscle types in space in parallel with Earth's slow muscles can affect position and ability to stand, are the most vulnerable to weakening, due to micro-gravity. However, on Earth, all research says that the fast muscles disappear first, at age, disease, etc.

SUMMARY

1G – Sleep > Muscle-specific addiction

0G – Sleep > Muscle independence

Untrained or aging muscles

It is natural that the muscles in space begin to weaken rapidly after launching when gravity is missing. The fact is that the increasing rate of space with a lack of gravity is an ongoing process in people who are untrained, in illness or with increasing age. Elderly people get the same result in the end, because the muscles need training in space as on earth. Missing daily activities that go to work, on stairs, shopping, muscle activation becomes too low and often not enough. Self-training in addition to the usual tasks has been shown by research to strengthen an aging body. The muscle strength blooms between the ages of twenty to forty and if you have a work that needs muscle strength, your body and muscles will grow to provide that service. And the opposite; your muscles will shrink due to lack of work, but it is a fine line between healthy work or excessive. More and more reports show training later in life is beneficial for everyday life and if a habit of exercising can continue through life is much gained. Independence and freedom later in life are some benefits from an active life. The cost in the world is increasing due to lack of movement. Not to mention the young people today are bred with mobile and computer, which makes it even more important to activate the young generation in order not to get galloping expenses in the future. A paradox: It is predicted that the young generation will receive most of the centenarians in modern times. A strategy for the elderly in society will be a hot spot for years to come.

With a decrease in hormones with age, many functions decrease. One of the most important features is sleep. Without a doubt, sleep can be the most important feature of humans, such as breathing and nutrition. Without oxygen, food and lack of sleep, survival is small in the long run.

Sometimes sedentary individuals reduce muscle mass and strength gradually after the age of 40. Age-related loss of skeletal muscle and function are risk factors for osteoporosis and fractures. Researchers found a close link to the Mediterranean diet was significantly associated with greater fat-free mass and explosive bone force, indicating the benefits of the Mediterranean diet to prevent loss of muscle mass.

SARCOPENIA

The medical word for a lost muscle mass is Sarcopenia. 25% of 65+ year-olds were affected and 60% of 80+ year-olds had these symptoms. The loss of skeletal muscle mass, strength and function with age contributes to risk factors for sarcopenia, weakness, osteoporosis, fractures and mortality. Sarcopenia is a well-established fact due to aging. Weakened physical function is increased twice in individuals with low muscle strength, which is a prediction for type 2 diabetes, cardiovascular and morbidity and low quality of life.

Consequences of SARKOPENIA:

- Reduced resting energy
- Decreased insulin sensitivity
- Reduced muscle strength and bulk
- Increase the risk of physical disability and falls
- Increase the risk of mortality

Cases for the elderly who have not trained significantly over the years increase the risk of fractures noticeably and it is not uncommon to see women with hip fractures at age 80 who have fallen into the apartment. The significant of this injury, unlike my own, rehab training begins almost immediately and therefore a good basic physics increase the prospects for a rapid improvement.

In early life as a young adult, with muscle growth and adult life tries to maintain peak, but older fighters to minimize muscle loss. Muscle mass and strength are more achievable when having type 2 fibers and practicing mixed training late in life.

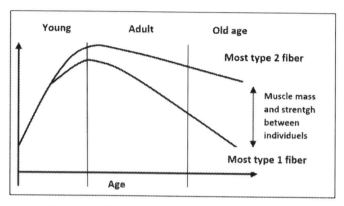

Figure 2 the span of muscle strength

Studies have shown that low strength in the hand grip is associated with cardiac metabolic risk and mortality. The overall muscle strength is associated with metabolic syndrome, but some researchers still say that the measurement of lower and upper body strength is a better prediction for health than hand grip strength. Researchers found that bone muscle strength was associated with an increased likelihood of metabolic syndrome. Experimental strength training supports the thesis that increased muscle strength reduces cardiometabolic risk. In fact, several strength training trials have shown clinical relevance and improvements in glycemic status and blood pressure in adults.

Muscle strength and mass are mostly highly correlated, but the relationship between low muscle mass and potency associated with mortality has been investigated. Certain thigh size was not strongly related to mortality, but showing muscle strength as a marker of muscle quality is more important than the quantity when assessing the risk of death. Grip strength gave risk assessments like those for thigh strength. For some people, those born with muscle mass (type 2 fibers) have some benefit. This group of people certainly has stronger muscle status in life, but if training fails, strength disappears faster than mass, which the studies reflected. Many analyze support that muscle strength is an important factor in health outcomes in men. Men with low muscle strength are more likely to show metabolic symptoms and increased cortisol levels. The presence of three or more of the following symptoms can predict age-related and alarming signs:

- Accidental weight loss, 4.5 kg in one year
- Self-reported fatigue
- Weakness in the dominant grip strength
- Slow walking speed
- Slow physical activity

HORMONES AND DECREASING MUSCLES

Testosterone plays a key role in the development of male reproductive tissues such as testicles and prostate, as well as promoting secondary sexual properties, such as increased muscle, bone mass and growth of body hair. Testosterone's effects on muscle strength and physical function in older men have been inconsistent, researchers say; its effects on muscle strength and fatigue have not been studied. To determine the effects of testosterone secretion for 3 years in older men, muscle strength, force and physical function were studied through stairwell, leg press and chest pressure exercises. The result shows significantly greater improvements in stairwell, muscle mass and force.

Low levels of important hormones have a key role in the age process of humans:

- Low testosterone
- Low growth hormone GH> Low IGF-1
- Increased cortisol

GH is a growth hormone that stimulates growth, cell reproduction in humans and is secreted into the anterior wings of the anterior pituitary gland. The Low growth hormone increase the concentration of glucose and free fatty acids, also stimulates the production of IGF-1. IGF-1 is mainly secreted by the liver as a result of growth hormone stimulation. IGF-I is important for both regulation of normal physiology and is increased by protein intake in humans regardless of total calorie consumption. IGF-1 stimulates body growth and has growth-promoting effects on almost every cell in the body, especially skeletal muscle, bone, nerves and skin.

SUMMARY

Experimental strength training supports the thesis that increased muscle strength improves cardiometabolic risk.

***

Muscle strength and mass are mostly highly correlated, but showing muscle strength as a marker of muscle quality is more important than the quantity when assessing the risk of death.

***

Factors known to cause variation in the levels of growth hormone and IGF-1 in the circulation include: Exercise status, stress levels, nutritional level and body index (BMI).

***

Men with low muscle strength are more likely to show metabolic symptoms and increased cortisol levels.

***

Measurement of lower and upper body strength is a better health prerequisite than hand grip strength.

***

Researchers found low bone muscle strength was associated with an increased likelihood of metabolic syndrome.

***

Muscle mass and strength are more achievable when having Type 2 muscles and practicing mixed training late in life.

***

Myokines

Researchers have shown that the volume of the anterior hippocampus increased by 2% in response to aerobic exercise in a randomized controlled study of 120 older adults. The authors also summarize several previously established research results related to exercise and brain function. Aerobic exercise increases the degree of gray and white matter in the anterior forehead of older adults. Exercise increases brain volume and hemoperfusion in the hippocampus. Increased hippocampal volume is associated with higher serum levels of BDNF, a mediator of neurogenesis (the formation of neurons). New research shows that skeletal muscles can produce and express cytokines belonging to different families. A myokine is one of several hundred cytokines or other small proteins that are produced and released by muscle cells in response to muscle contractions. Skeletal muscles express and release myokines in the circulation.

Exercise-induced benefits are well known to prevent the deleterious effects of proinflammatory adipokins secreted from fat cells, to control fat and glucose metabolism, with multiple functions.

Receptors for myokines are found in muscle, fat, liver, pancreas, bone, heart, and brain cells. The site of these receptors explains that myokines have several functions and they are involved in exercise-related metabolic changes. Different types of muscle fibers emit different myokines during contraction, which explains that variety of exercise types. Particularly aerobic exercise and muscle contraction with strength training can offer different myokine-induced benefits.

Exercise-induced myokines can be the potential candidates to provide beneficial effects by stimulating metabolic pathways, improving glucose uptake, improving fat oxidation and regulating skeletal muscle regeneration.

IRISIN

Irisin is commonly referred to as the "training hormone" as it is released during moderate aerobic endurance when cardiorespiratory systems are in operation and the muscles are used. The results from several studies suggest that the iris content was increased in rodents and humans after exercise. Therefore, irisin has potential as a therapeutic agent. Study shows that irisin combats fat with two steps.

1. Enable genes and convert white fat cells into browns, which continue to burn energy upon completion of exercise.
2. By inhibiting the formation of fatty tissue.

INTERLEUKIN-6

Aerobic exercise induces a systemic protein activation of the cell. The exercise-induced increase in plasma IL-6 occurs in an exponential manner and the peak IL-6 level is reached at the end of the training or shortly thereafter. A combination of intensity and duration determines the size of the exercise-induced increase in plasma level. IL-6 was discovered as a myokine because it increases up to 100 times in the circulation during physical exercise and also appears to have systemic effects on the liver, adipose tissue and immune system. Some studies show that strength training is not associated with a larger increase in plasma IL-6 in exercise involving muscle breakdown and contractions. Which clearly shows that muscle breakdown is not required to provoke an increase in plasma IL-6 during exercise.

INTERLEUKIN-15

IL-15 is a newly discovered growth factor that is strongly expressed in the skeletal muscle. IL-15 has been shown to have anabolic effects on the skeletal muscles and appears to play a role in the reduction of fat mass, but also in the growth of skeletal muscle fibers has been presented as a hypothesis. IL-15 can stimulate differentiated muscle cells and muscle fibers to accumulate increased amounts of contracting proteins in the skeletal muscle. After strength training, the IL-15 increases protein content in plasma.

FIBROBLAST GROWTH FACTOR-21

FGF-21, an endocrine hormone, plays an important role in the development of metabolic regulation by regulating glucose and fat metabolism. FGF-21 is expressed in peripheral tissues, such as white adipose tissue, liver, pancreas and skeletal muscle. FGF-21 levels increase under starvation and ketogenic conditions.

AMPK

AMPK is a critical regulator of cell energy homeostasis. This is why it is no surprise that it is also closely linked to the regulation of biochemical pathways that affect cell survival and profiling. AMPK activation:

- Fat oxidation
- Cell profiling
- Glycos transport

New discoveries may suggest a direct AMPK role to increase blood supply to muscle cells. During a single exercise session, AMPK allows the contracting muscle cells to adapt by increasing glucose uptake.

BDNF-SLEEP GRAIL

BDNF, a signal protein in the central nervous system, is expressed most and to a large extent in the brain. So far, many studies have suggested that BDNF may play a role not only in central metabolic pathways but also as a metabolic regulator of the skeletal muscle. Many studies showed that BDNF increased in human skeletal muscle after exercise and is produced by the release of contracting muscles in the blood circulation. BDNF appears in skeletal muscle to improve fat oxidation. Muscle activation through exercise also contributes to an increase in BDNF secretion in the brain. A positive effect of BDNF on neuronal function has been noted in several studies.

Strength training is a popular form of exercise that is recommended by national health organizations. However, individual response to strength training has been reported. Some people significantly increased BDNF while others did not, which helps to individualize exercise recipes to optimize results according to many researchers.

Animal studies reduced BDNF levels following chronic stress. Serum BDNF levels decreased in stress-related depressive disease. The great stress response system HPA facilitates adaptation to stress.

BDNF is a biomarker of impaired memory and general cognitive function in aging women. Low circulating BDNF levels were recently shown to be an independent and robust biomarker of mortality risk. Studies have shown that physical exercise can increase circulating BDNF levels. In humans, a BDNF release was observed from the brain at rest and increased 2- to 3-fold during exercise.

BDNF plays an important role in neuronal survival and growth; it is extensively expressed in CNS, intestine and other tissues. Reduced levels of BDNF are associated with nerve degenerative diseases such as:

- Parkinson's disease

- Alzheimer's disease
- Multiple sclerosis

BDNF has been shown to regulate neuronal development and plays a role in learning and memory. In addition, it is well established that BDNF plays a role in controlling body weight and energy hemostasis. New evidence identifies BDNF as a player not only in central metabolism but also in regulating energy metabolism in peripheral organs. An increase in BDNF derived from physical activity is believed to increase adult nerve and synapse formation and contribute to cognitive benefits and reduced psychiatric symptoms.

The circulating level of BDNF is reduced in patients with major depression and type 2 diabetes. Training increases BDNF production and researchers suggest that endurance training promotes brain health. The research and discussion has been intensive over BDNF health benefits in humans. Observations of decreased serum levels in patients with neuropsychiatric disorders have highlighted BDNF as a biomarker. However, animal experiments have shown positive results between blood serum levels and hippocampal BDNF levels in rats and pigs. In addition, there was significant positive correlation between frontal cortex and hippocampal BDNF levels in mice.

Also studies on yoga and increased BDNF. Subjects proved to be associated with reductions in self-reported anxiety and depression. The increased BDNF level observed is a potential mediator between meditative methods and brain health.

BDNF AND SLEEP

BDNF plays a role in sleep regulation. People suffering from insomnia showed significantly reduced BDNF levels in blood serum. One study showed that the interaction between stress and sleep affects BDNF levels, which demonstrates an important role in the pathogenesis of stress-related mental disorders. In addition, insomnia is often observed in many stress-related diseases. The neurotrophin hypothesis (growth factor-small proteins) is based on these properties and suggests that stress-related mental disorders are the result of stress-induced reduction of BDNF expression. Although a majority of studies have concentrated on specifying the role of BDNF in depression.

There is many evidence that BDNF expression is reduced by perceived mental stress and that a lack of neurotrophic support leads to major depression. Recently, for the first time, a relationship between BDNF and insomnia was reported. BDNF plays a key role in the pathophysiology of stress-related mood disorders.

The results of the experiments strongly support the supposed causal link between BDNF and SWA regulation. This result indicates that BDNF is involved in triggering the sleep-regulating deep sleep waves observed after both spontaneous alertness and sleep disturbance. Sleep can be affected by exercise, as physical activity alters the endocrine, autonomic nervous system (ANS).

A single exercise exercise increases the amount of subsequent SWS, slow sleep waves, according to study. Training just before you lay down creates for some a stress effect that can reduce the amount of subsequent SWS. This effect may be greater sometimes aerobic exercise with oxygen-demanding exercise late at night. However, the antidepressant effects of exercise have recently been studied well and improved mood that can be attributed to a BDNF increase that can be attributed to exercise can indirectly improve sleep quality.

The study examined BDNF in the hippocampus caused by sleep deprivation and regulated the abnormal expression of BDNF caused by sleep disturbances in the short and long term. Synaptic activity in the hippocampus facilitated the onset of BDNF in the hippocampus.

SUMMARY

Sleep is affected by exercise, as physical activity affects endocrine, autonomic nervous system (ANS).

***

Synaptic activity in the hippocampus facilitated the onset of BDNF.

***

Physical exercise increases circulating BDNF levels in humans. BDNF release was observed from the brain at rest and increased 2- to 3-fold during exercise.

***

People suffering from insomnia showed significantly reduced BDNF levels in blood serum.

***

A single exercise exercise increases the amount of subsequent SWS, slow sleep waves, deep sleep.

***

The Neurotrophin hypothesis, growth factors, suggests that stress-related mental disorders are the result of stress-induced reduction of BDNF expression.

***

Also studies on yoga and increased BDNF. The increased level observed is a potential mediator between meditative methods and brain health, according to researchers.

***

Reduced levels of BDNF are associated with neurodegenerative diseases such as: Parkinson's disease, Alzheimer's disease, Multiple sclerosis

***

Muscle types

The basic problem for many people is the lack of ability to rest, you feel excited and not ready for sleep. Here is an important task to solve. We have six hundred muscles in the body and for some reason they cannot relax on command. Even if you do not use your body with physical work at work, muscle becomes stiff. In addition, stress moments also add to muscle stiffness. With a larger proportion of narrow muscles, the body is created for a higher stress level, but it can also mean that it becomes more difficult to turn off the stress when needed. There are some muscle features to consider:

- React to stimuli
- Ability to shorten
- Ability to extend during draw
- Return to original shape and length by time

Even if you just have a nice walk or go out with your dog, you do something and use a lot of muscle. By using muscles, you retain the following features:

- Movement
- Posture
- Heat

The legs provide posture and structural support for the body. The muscles allow the body to move, but also provides protection for the body's internal organs. The muscles are attached to the bone by tendons, ligaments and cartilage. They vary in shape and size and serve many different purposes. For the most part, they control the larger muscles movement, but all muscles share the same basic structure at the microscopic level. The muscle consists of bundles of muscle fibers. The muscle fibers, in turn, are composed of thousands of cellular threads that can be contracted, relaxed and extended. The cell wires are organized in repeated subunits along its length. This subunit is called sarcoma. Each sarcoma is made of overlapping thick and thin filaments / wires consisting of contractile proteins, mainly actin and myosin. When a muscle is contracted, actin is drawn along the myosin toward the center of the sarcoma until actin and myosin filaments are completely overlapped.

The rest of the sarcoplasm includes:

- Mitochondria, energy Type 1 fiber
- Lipids
- Glycogen, energy type 2 fiber
- T-tubules

The T-tubules are responsible for conducting electrical signals from the cell surface to the inner regions of muscle fibers. The electrical signals performed by the T-tubule stimulate the sarcoplasm to release calcium. When an electrical signal reaches the neuro-muscular junction, deep within the muscle fibers, the signal stimulates the flow of calcium, causing the thick and thin myofilaments to slide over each other. When this occurs, it causes the sarcoma to shorten, generating power. When all the sarcomas in the muscle are shortened at once, it results in a contraction of all muscle fibers. When more muscle fibers are recruited by the central nervous system, the stronger is the force generated by muscular contraction.

Release of calcium > Contraction

MAIN TYPES OF MUSCLE FIBERS

The human skeletal muscle contains two main types: Type 1 and Type 2, the latter with normally three complementary muscle fibers a, b, and x. Some researchers and physiologists indicate an additional subtype Type 2c.

- **TYPE 1 - Slow fiber**
- **TYPE 2a - First fast fibers**
- **TYPE 2b - Middle fast fiber**
- **TYPE 2x - Fastest fiber**

The fast fibers are recruited late. They are used for short-term intensive activity and for transporting heavy loads and are specialized in anaerobic metabolism. A common type 2 muscle is Vastus lateralis (thigh), which contains more than 50 % type 2 fibers. Under extreme conditions, type 2X fibers activate as the last resources.

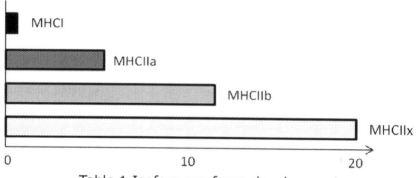

Table 1 Isoformers force development

Regardless of fiber size, MHC (Myosin Heavy Chain) 2a fibers produce 6 times more power, and fibers with MHC 2x produce up to 20 times more power than MHC I fibers.

Limiting the range of motion can create an imbalance in the muscle. The muscles can be shortened by postural adaptation and activated by spasm or contraction. Stiffness limits the range of motion and can create an imbalance in the muscle. When it comes to stretching, muscle tension is usually inversely related to length:

The muscle tension is usually inversely related to length:

- Reduced muscle tension> Increased muscle length
- Increased muscle tension> Decreased muscle length

TYP 1 FIBER

Type 1 fibers are thus slow to contraction, but they are also durable and can easily withstand muscle work for a long time. They are durable because they contain more mitochondria, the cell's power plant, than the fast fibers and can therefore produce more energy. Type 1 fibers are also smaller in diameter and have increased capillary blood flow, which provides more oxygen and remove more waste products from the muscle fibers, which also reduces their "fatigue". Physiologists refer to them as slow oxidative (Slow-Oxidative, SO) fibers. If a muscle is gradually loaded, the slow fibers are first recruited, after which the muscle is recruited the strongest are recruited. They are used for long-term activity at a low level. A common type 1 muscle is the delta muscle, shoulder, which has a greater amount of slow muscle than fast

Description	Typ I
Kontraction	Slow
Utmattning	Slow
Activity	Aerobic
Duration	Hours
Power	Weak
Mitochondria	Many
Capillary	Many
Testosteron	Low
Cortisol	High
Color	Dark red
Diameter	Narrow

Type 1 fibers must take the big challenge of keeping the body running and performing the most fundamental movements in life. Type 1 fiber that remains when we get older, to the end, and it is an oxygen demanding process with many mitochondria and capillaries. Characteristic of narrow persons with high cortisol value, which normally reflects the stress threshold.

Table 2 Description of Typ1-muscle fiber.

Type 1 fibers work for hours, with low strength and high cortisol levels.

TYP 2-FIBER

Many studies make it more hopeful for those with weaker sleep engine. Could it be a truth; the better sleep - the fewer Type 1 muscles you have. It is more difficult to move from Type 1 muscle to Type 2; compared to if you are created with strong muscles since birth. It will need a little effort to make a muscle shift, but on the other hand it is much easier to maintain a stronger muscle status once it has been achieved.

Description	Typ 2 a	Typ 2 b
Contraction time	Moderat-Fast	Very fast
Fatigue	Moderat	Fast
Activity	Middle anaerob	Anaerob
Duration	< 30 min	< 1 min
Power	Middle	Very high
Mitokondrier	Middle	Few
Capillarities	Many	Few
Testosteron	High	Very High
Cortisol	Low	Very Low
Color	Red	Light red
Diameter	Middle-thick	Thick

Table 3 Fiber description of Typ 2a och 2b

The table above describes two fiber types of the faster variety. The fastest x-fiber is not described here. It has a fast operation in seconds. Using all three fast muscle types should be a sign to turn a weak sleep engine. Working with the interval of a few seconds to half an hour you get both fitness and muscles. To peak the training with the strong Type 2x fiber provides good breeding ground for an increased testosterone level.

Exercise habits have a direct impact on the composition of the muscle fibers. Type 1 muscle fibers favor higher cortisol levels and type 2 muscle fibers favor higher testosterone. A poor testosterone-to-cortisol ratio provides a catabolic state (muscle waste). Endurance training not only produces cortisol and inhibits testosterone, but it also provides a shift from Type 2 to Type 1 muscle fibers.

It is particularly important to use lifelong exercise systems that can suppress the age-related decrease in muscle fibers, especially for the type 2 muscle fibers. Importantly, only strength-trained individuals exhibited improved fast muscle strength and increased muscle fiber size compared to non-training elderly. Persistent elderly people use a larger proportion of type I muscle fibers than untrained people. Type 2 muscle fibers were elevated in the trained elderly, but not in endurance-trained individuals compared to the untrained, which suggests that resistance training is superior to endurance training to delay age-related loss in muscle mass. It is particularly effective in counteracting the decrease in type 2 fiber area normally observed with high age.

SUMMARY

Type 2 fiber is driven by testosterone, a building hormone.

***

A short activation Type 2 fiber to balance the deactivated Type 1 fiber.

***

Older men generally have significant muscle atrophy with selective loss of the fast type II fiber.

***

The sum of all trained type 2 fibers indicates a low cortisol level.

***

Exercising calves and thighs is perhaps the best sleep advice, since a redistribution of these muscle fibers can have a significant impact on better sleep.

General training advice

A program with regular and versatile training in addition to everyday activities applies to maintaining physical fitness and health for most individuals. In addition to exercising regularly, there are health benefits to reducing at the same time the total time spent on sedentary activities. Short moments of standing and physical activity between periods of sedentary activity are also recommended for physically active adults.

We all have different experiences of physical activity, but it is never too late to regain lost years. The optimum is to maintain a physical lifestyle from the early years. Physical activity can be described as:

- Sedentary; no activity in the last three months
- Moderately active; Leisure activity or walking, jogging or running ≤ 15 km per week
- Highly active; walked, jogging or running> 15 km per week

Physical inactivity plays a central role in age-related reduction of muscle strength, an important component of the process leading to disability. Physical activity can therefore affect muscle strength during adulthood and affect the rate of decline with aging. Strong evidence shows that good muscle strength in middle age protects against disability in later life, highlighting the importance of maintaining muscle strength through life.

Physical inactivity plays a central role in age-related reduction of muscle strength, an important component of the process leading to disability. Physical activity can therefore affect muscle strength during adulthood and affect the rate of decline with aging. Strong evidence shows that good muscle strength in middle age protects against disability in later life, highlighting the importance of maintaining muscle strength through life.

Physical activity includes all forms of activity. Different types of exercise are as follows:

- Aerobics (walking, swimming, group training)
- Anaerobic (sprint, shorter intensive exercise)
- Isotonic (weight training)

Popular and with a rising trend, group training is in fitness facilities. Different workouts with leaders attract more and more and it benefits those who do not want to decide what to do for them self. The advantage of group training is to be together and the gym companies often have a variety of training disciplines to choose from, from yoga to mother training. Usually there is also a gym that is a complement to group training. Targeting your training to fit your own body and function is part of the training experience for most people.

Despite the health effects of training in some form, research shows that only an estimated 50% of all people who initiate an exercise program continue training for more than 6 months.

Athletic aspirations or extensive plans for a lifetime of appropriate physical activity are usually indicated by researchers to:

- 4-6 times a week
- 30 minutes during most days of the week

Choose a lifetime activity or vary several types of activity. In particular, choose an activity that is fun and anyone uses most of the muscles, raises the heart rate and can be durable for 20 minutes or longe

RESISTANCE TRAINING

Resistance or strength training should be a complement rather than a replacement for aerobic exercise. Resistance training increases muscle strength and is often recommended by major health organizations to improve health and exercise. The literature shows that the most important contributor to the loss of muscle function with aging is a quantitative loss of muscle mass. Elderly men generally have significant muscle atrophy with selective loss of the fast Type 2 fiber. In order to prevent large losses in peak force with aging, it is important to reduce the muscle wasting and loss of function of the Type 2 fiber.

Research can sometimes show varying results, but results strengthen the evidence that aerobic exercise and strength training are different physiological stimuli with respect to concentration of growth factors. Exercise can be conducted in a variety of ways and in addition, the effect can be different as muscle composition varies from person to person.

The muscle strength is inverted and independently associated with mortality from all causes and cancers in men, write researchers. They claim that it can be possible to reduce severe mortality among men by promoting regular strength training involving the major muscle groups in the upper body and lower body two or three days a week.

Lifting weights or using strength training machines strengthens the legs, especially if you practice all major muscle groups in the legs, arms and torso. A qualified trainer, training specialist or therapist is important for instructing and controlling exercise programs. Joining a gym or training facility is a good way to start, as these facilities provide access to trainers who can advise on suitable techniques.

Resistance training is recommended by most health promotion organizations for effects such as:

- Strength
- Muscle mass
- Bone mineral density
- Functional capacity
- Preventive rehabilitation

Resistance training is about giving some kind of resistance to the contracting muscles to stimulate the body to increase strength. Several types of equipment are used for resistance training. Suitable resistance tools: hand weights, elastic resistance, machines.

Strength or resistance training is very important to improve functionality and reduce the risk of injury. As people age, it reduces muscle tissue, more from lack of use than from aging itself. Regularly performing some type of resistance training is absolutely necessary.

Frequency, duration and intensity of activity should be individually tailored to personal satisfaction and purpose. General advice on strength training, using free weights or standard equipment, is usually stated:

- 2-3 times a week
- 8-10 training sets
- 10-15 repetitions per set

Including arms, shoulders, chest, back, hips and legs and performed with moderate intensity. Strength exercises tend to supplement aerobic exercise, but the development of muscle tone and strengthening of body muscles is more important as adult's age.

Repetitions are a science in itself and everyone who strengthens regularly has own philosophy on the number of reps, which depends on the purpose of the exercise and exercise status. Classic number of reps is 8 for regular training. For beginners, about 15-30 repetitions can be done and perceived efforts should only be moderate or somewhat difficult.

Strength training is a slow process, so it should be started at a low level and should be gradually built up over several months and years. For each exercise, you choose weights or set the machine so that the muscle becomes tired after 10-15 repetitions. In a completely new exercise, more reps can be used to "teach" the muscle exercise. Then 15-30 reps can be used. Gradually add more weight when the muscles become stronger. The weight should not be increased more than 10% per week, as greater increases may increase the risk of injury.

Having strong muscles is somewhat beneficial and is better for everyday life. A strong body and strong heart can improve your status later in life. Early in life, if you start exercising and continue in adulthood, much is gained. Checking strong legs for your sleep list should be number one and a rule for the modern man.

Exercising legs, what and thighs should be on the agenda in the gym a couple of times a week. Exercising the inner and outer calf muscles is perhaps the best sleep advice, as a redistribution of these muscle fibers can have a significant impact on better sleep. Train your calves, preferably with easier resistance. Start with many resp. and at some point breaks off with fewer or less, and heavier weights. The times that no leg training has been performed can advantageously be used for bed and thighs before bedtime. More on this topic in later chapters.

Developing and maintaining aerobic endurance, joint flexibility and muscle strength is important in a comprehensive exercise program, especially when people age.

Several studies suggest that relatively small amounts of physical activity show significant reductions in mortality and improved health outcomes among participants compared to sedentary. Some authors have suggested a physical activity threshold may be necessary for optimal health.

SUMMARY

Studies indicate that relatively small amounts of physical activity show significant reductions in mortality and improved health outcomes among participants compared to sedentary.

***

Fitness??? training generally induces a fast to slow fiber-type transition, with a reduction of type 2a fibers, and a maintenance or increase of type 1 fibers.

***

Physical activity affects muscle strength during adulthood and affects the rate of muscle strength decline with aging.

***

Strong evidence shows good muscle strength in middle age protects against disability in later life, highlighting the importance of maintaining muscle strength throughout life.

***

Research has shown the current evidence-based basis for prescribing training as a medicine in the treatment of 26 different diseases.

***

A short boost of medium-strength Type 2 fiber gives more of the short sleep waves, deep sleep.

***

Strength training induces a robust increase in circulating BDNF and which affects brain health and lowers the aurosal level.

***

Leg training – Sleep training

Functional training of the whole body. Strengthen the body from the natural movement pattern. For the substance in this book, sleep - Bone training should be intensified for some time to come until your sleep reaches a higher level. Important with pump and strength. Here are some suggestions.

- **Strength training - Specific Type 2x fiber**
- **Pump training - Specific Type 2b fiber**
- **Oxygen training - Specific Type 2a fiber**

Strength training – Max sessions with few repetitions increases maximul strength.

Pump Training - Volume Pass with many repetitions increase the muscle area in the legs and also increase the pulse, the heart may work. Volume training with short rest periods gives weak aerobic function training. Volume training twice a week provides a good boost for increased volume, and a good breeding ground for increasing strength over time, so as not to break with increased weight.

Oxygen training - Fitness pass more heart training, but with focus on middle distance 5-20 minutes activity divided into two passes. The pass is no amount training, but should increase the pulse noticeably, once or twice a week. Fitness training generally induces a fast to slow fiber type transition with a Type 2a fiber reduction and a Type 1 fiber increase or maintenance, to be avoided. A bit quicker and shorter passports will endorse the purpose better.

FOUR-DAYS program to increase sleep quality. The days can of course be changed to fit your own schedule. The important thing with the whole program is to perform the leg training and if the outcome is the intended one, the schedule can then be changed to fit the whole body.

WEEKLY SCHEDULE

Monday
Varming up 5 min - Cycling, running, cross, rowing
Pump Training-leg
Stretch when needed

Tuesday
Varming up 5 min - Cycling, running, cross, rowing
Oxygen Training
Stretch when needed

Wednesday
Varming up 5 min - Cycling, running, cross, rowing
Free training.
Stretch when needed

Thursday
Varming up 5 min - Cycling, running, cross, rowing
Max training legs
Stretch when needed

1. LEGPRESS

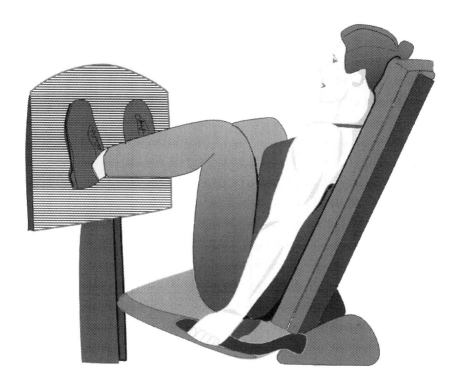

Figure 3. Leg press

MASHINE; thigh, gluteus and back
Pump 30 reps * 3, Light weight
Rest 1-2 min between reps
Alt. Reps 30, 25, 20

Strength 5-10 reps * 3, heavy weight
Rest 1-2 minutes between reps, or as long as you need to cope with the number of reps.

2. LEG KICK, FRONT OF THIGH AND SATE?

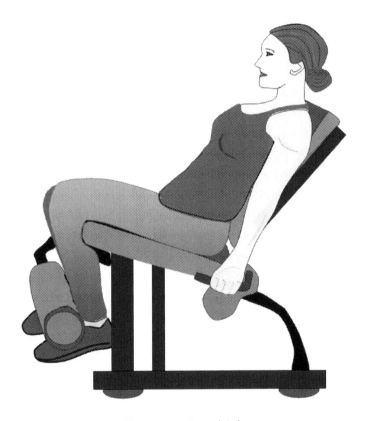

Figure 4. Leg kick

MASHINE; Front of thigh and gluteus
Kick up until the legs are straight. Adjustable starting position. The farther towards the seat, the further up the thigh you work with.

Pump 30 reps * 3, light weight
Rest 1-2 minutes between reps, or as long as you need to cope with the number of reps.
Alt. Reps 30, 25, 20

Strength 5-15 reps*3, heavy weight
Rest1-2 min between reps

3. LEG CURL

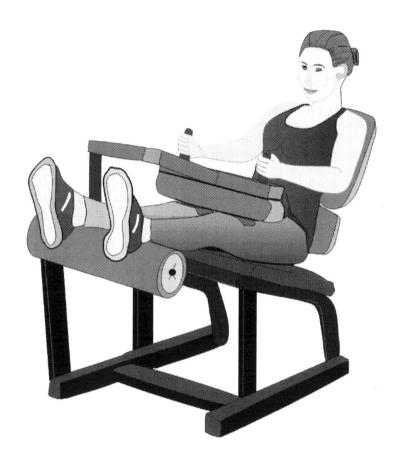

Figure 5. Leg curl

MASHINE; back of thigh and gluteus.
Sitting. Alt lying on stomach

Pump 30 reps * 3, Lätt vikt
Rest 1-2 minutes between reps, or as long as you need to cope with the number of reps.

Strength 5-15 reps*3, heavy weight
Rest 1-2 min between reps.
Start with straight legs; press the heels straight down, as far as it will go.

4. SQUATS

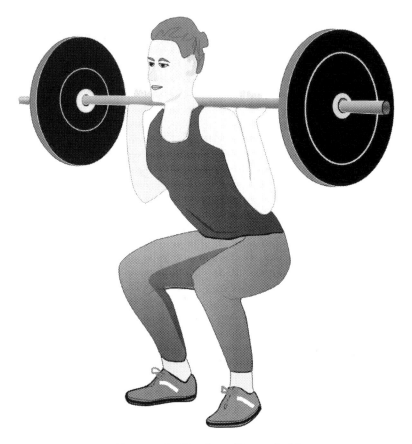

Figure 6. Sqats with weight

FREE WEIGHT OR MASHINE; thigh, gluteus, back
Pump 30 reps * 3, light weight
Rest 1-2 minutes between reps, or as long as you need to cope with the number of reps.

Strenght 5-10 reps*3, heavy weight
Rest 1-2 min between reps.
Versatile training. Start with just the bar if you've never done this exercise before. There are also machines where the rod is fixed, and then no balance is required.

5. CALF PRESS

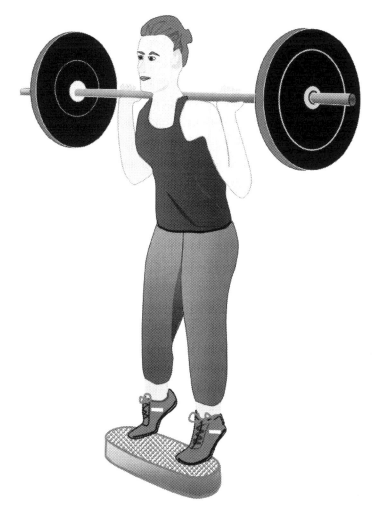

Figure 7 Calf press with weight

MASHINE OR FREE ROD; interior and inferior calf
Pump 30 reps * 3, Light weight
Rest 1-2 min between reps

Strenght 5-15 reps * 3, heavy weight
Rest 1-2 min between reps.

FREE STANDING – LIGHT LEG-PROGRAM
1. Stationäry outcome; thigh, calf and gluteus

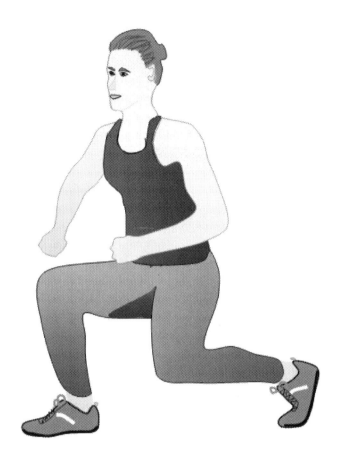

Figure 8. Stationary outcome, easy program

**Without weight
50 reps * 3, rest 60 sek**

**With weight, hantle
10-20 reps*3, rest 60 sek**

The outcome technique is the same as the activation exercise before going to bed, but with a focus on muscle building.

2. Squats; calf, thigh and gluteus

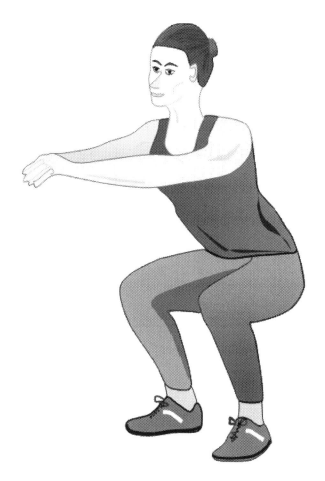

Figure 9. Squats, easy program

Without weight
50 reps * 3, rest 60 sek

With hand weight/hantle
20 reps*3, rest 60 sek

Squats technique is the same as activation exercise before bed, but with focus on muscle building.

3. Toe press; foot and calf

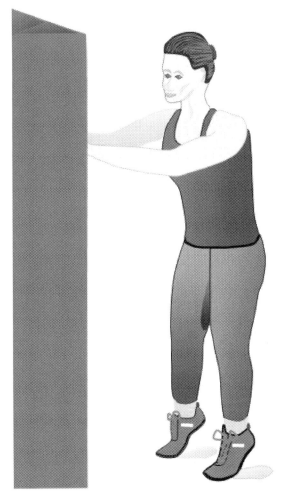

Figure 10. Toe press, easy program

Without weight
50 reps * 3, rest 60 sek

With hand weight
20 reps*3, rest 60 sek

Toe press technique is the same activation exercise before bed, but with focus on muscle building.

Activation of Type 2 fibers

Since I started stretching 30 years ago and my own studies of sleep / stretching, my own perception has gone in the opposite direction. A direction that does not go against the stretching philosophy, but is a supplement. Activating the muscles before bedtime may not all buy at first, especially as stretching suggests the opposite. This section of my sleep theory points to type 2 fibers as part of the sacred grail of sleep. Stretching and activation provide a perfect breeding ground for better sleep. According to medical facts, there is one variant of Type 1 fibers and several of Type 2 fibers, which means that the scale from the slim fiber to the stronger is transient. From the oxygen-driving Type 1 fiber to the opposite, a smoth transition allows for gentle oxygen declining.

The research on muscle-related genes and myokines is in its infancy, but is becoming increasingly intense every year. Expectations in this field promise good for the future. Examination of the BDNF beneficial effects of exercise is varied and most of the evidence suggests that the effect is as great as oxygen-intensive exercise. However, there is research that shows that strength training also gives positive results. The results are expected to be rewritten in several ways in the future and perhaps show more benefits, which are not completely clear for the moment.

These 30 minutes after activation, when BDNF is secreted, provide a much-needed supplement of BDNF before bedtime. A quick Type 2 activation can provide just that addition.

Activating Type 2 muscles is of the highest priority, as it promotes health and better sleep. Strength and cardio training should be combined for best results, as the two different types of muscles require completely different training. The best result for sleep is a focus on the legs. The legs have the strongest and largest muscles in the body and also variations of Type 1 and Type 2. The four-headed thigh muscle consists of 55% Type 2 fibers and the inner calf muscle Soleus consists of 65% Type 1 fibers, which makes the perfect balance between two types are activation and stretching.

The alpha arrhythmia's gate to sleep provides a relaxed drowsiness that increases the chances of activating sleep hormones via the para-sympathetic nervous system. It is very difficult to fall asleep when the sympathetic nervous system (day system) pumps into the body. A good sleeper has a natural sleep switch, which is not usually the case for a person with a weak sleep engine. However, it should be said that insomnia has many causes and may arise from obsticals that have to be reviewed first.

A well-trained body, with an even distribution of different forms of exercise is preferable. The stress hormone cortisol is bound to the narrower muscles, and it is important to raise the testosterone that is bound to the Type 2 muscle. A good all-round exercise a few times a week, focusing primarily on skeletal muscles in the legs raises the level of constructive hormones.

It may seem that exercise should not be conducted shortly before sleep, but this exercise is not to be regarded as training even if you perform a muscle work. In order to balance the part of the body that contains the most muscle volume and strength, muscle activation is what is needed for the Type 2 fibers. However, it is a delicate difference in activation and training. The meaning of this sleep exercise, is that it should only be run for 10-60 seconds and only activate Type 2b fibers, which then forms an anaerobic activity and does not significantly increase heart activity. Start with the time interval that suits you. This exercise is suitable for performing if other training has not been conducted during the day.

ACTIVATING 1 – SQUATS

Thigh and glutesus muscles stand for the lifting force in this exercise, but most other muscles help to stabilize. Stomach and lower back maintain the lift. When lifting with weights, they are more important to stabilize the weight down to the legs. But this exercise is done without weights and for a while before going to bed. The exercise involves a brief activation of Type 2b muscles, which these two muscles represent most.

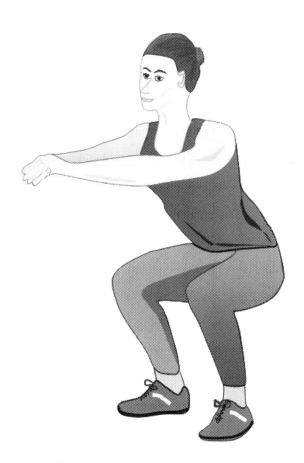

Figure 11. Activating - Squats.

EXECUTION

Squat down with your knees. The thigh should be in balance with the floor if it goes, but do the best you can. The important thing is to activate Type 2b and then it is necessary to try to get as far down and parallel to the floor. Bring your arms straight forward to balance your body. The exercise itself is to bring the body up 10 centimeters and back in several recurring movements. Important, only 10 centimeters, as activation of type 2 fibers is the purpose of the exercise.

The higher up the more type 1 fibers are activated. It can be difficult to get down parallel to the floor to begin with, but try to start with 45 degrees from the vertical. Note; this exercise requires good movement in the ankle. In the beginning, it may be good to grab a table edge with your hands to balance your body vertically, unless it just works to place your arms straight ahead. You are not supposed to be more energetic from this exercise, activation should only activate non-oxygen fibers. Since no weights are present, the exercise should only feel comfortable.

ACTIVATING 1B – STATIONARY OUTCOME

This exercise is a complementary exercise to the first, which is considered the more important of the two. Remember that all people are unique and therefore each exercise can be received differently. What feels good for a person can be perceived as the opposite of another.

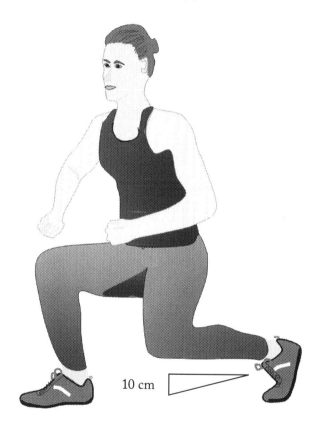

Figure 12 Activating – stationary outcome

Staionary outcome is a complex exercise also a bit more of a balancing exercise, because the legs are wide apart, forward and backward. Stationary outcomes are based on strength and stability in the legs, hip and calves.

EXECUTION

Don't confuse this exercise with a common outcome. Stand with both legs spaced forward and backward, the longer gaps between the legs, the more difficult to perform. Go down with your body until the back knee turns the floor, or as far as you can get. Repeat the exercise with short movements up and down. About 10 centimeters interval. Note that these two exercises should provide the most activation of Type 2b fibers and should not replace a real exercise of the day. However, it fits well if you have not trained legs during the day / evening.

ACTIVATING 2 – TOE PRESS

An important exercise with activation of the calf muscles. This exercise is the biggest contradiction, since it is mainly the deactivation of the calf muscles that is the most important, but that is mainly for the relaxation phase

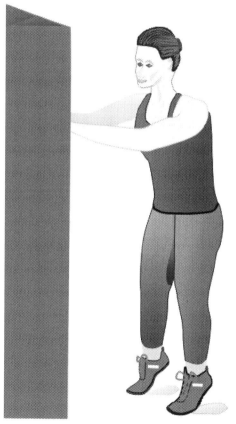

Figure 13. Activating – toe press

Activation is about the sleep phase and having strong calfs is a great advantage for good sleep. The calfs are small muscles and if one can convert some of the Type 1 fibers to Type 2, it is very much won.

EXECUTION

Stand with your legs slightly apart. Raise heels and arches so that only the toes remain on the floor. Use a door frame or chair back to balance. Start with 20 repetitions because it is not about training but only an activation phase. This exercise mostly activates the outer calf muscle, which has more Type 2 fibers than the inner one.

Type I Muscles And Deactivation

The purpose of this chapter is to introduce and lay a foundation for a better understanding of what stretching / deactivation can do for a stressed body. Also to show the most important concepts in a stretched muscle and why deactivation can help improve relaxation.

For many people, stretching is an important part practiced almost every day; when exercising, stretching is part of the daily exercise. Stretching is used at the beginning and end of the sessions to maintain muscle status and reduce stiffness in the muscle, no matter what the athlete is exercising. Of course, you do not need to be a top athlete to use stretching, but how many stretches regularly and how many tend to stretch before going to sleep? I mean, after a full working day, you do not need muscle relaxation! I think there is a large group of people who need regular stretching. For some, those with mostly soft muscles (type 2) and joints do not need stretching. The answer for these people can be more exercise / activation without stretching.

Stretching is a common activity used by sports practitioners, fitness practitioners, rehabilitation patients and anyone parti-cipating in an exercise program. When the pros and cons of stretching are known, the controversy about the best type of stretching for a particular target or outcome can still be found. Here, the current concepts of stretch interventions, summary and evidence relating to stretching used in both exercise and rehabilitation are described.

PROPRIOCEPTORS

The nerve endings that communicate all information about the muscle / skeleton system to the central nervous system are called proprioceptors. They discover changes in physical movement, position and tension. Proprioceptors are found in all nerve endings in joints, muscles and tendons. The proprioceptors read the muscles' status in work as a rest, which is of great importance for how the muscle tension affects a weak sleep engine. The readings of muscle tension of a proprioceptor, that is related to stretching, lies primarily between the tendons and the muscle fibers and is called the Golgis tendon organ. Muscle coils are the primary proprioceptors in the muscle.

Thus, there are two important biological properties to keep control of the muscles.

- Muscle spindle
- The Golgi tendon organ

MUSCLE SPINDLE

Muscle spindle is the sensory receptors in the muscle and is aligned parallel to extrafusive muscle fibers, consisting of three to twelve intrafusal muscle fibers, and primarily identifies the change in length of this muscle. That Information can be treated by the brain to determine the position of the body parts. The responses to the length of the muscle coils also play an important role in regulating the contraction of the muscles.

GOLGI TENDON ORGAN

Golgi tendon organ is a sensory receptor organ that lies between muscle and tendon. It gives the sensory part of the Golgi the tendon reflex, which is mainly for the muscle to not be overloaded and brake. Golgi senor also measures the tension at rest, which provides important information about current tension status.

Both of these muscle organs have important properties

for measuring the activity of the muscles and for the brain to have an accurate control. That means if there is tension and stiffness in large leg muscles, a signal is sent to the CNS from these organs. If there is muscle tension before going to bed, it may be more difficult to relax. If a bunch of muscles are tense, especially in the legs, the CNS receives a report that corresponds to the extent of the tense muscles. If you have a weak sleep engine and signals that correspond to tension in the muscles, it is more difficult to achieve Alfarytm. Remember, Type 1 fibers are cortisol-driven. When these narrow fibers become deactivated by stretching, the correct signals come to the CNS. A reaction that supports this reasoning is yawning spread through deactivation. Your deactivation organ is Golgi tendon organ.

STRETCH TECHNIQUES

There are normally three types of stretching described in the research literatures:

- Passive
- Static
- Dynamic

PASSIVE STRETCH

As the name indicates, the practitioner is passive throughout the stretching and entrusts the physical exercise to a second helping party. The practitioner can then be totally relaxed and get helped with stretching.

DYNAMIC STRETCH

Dynamic stretch is based on various movements that prepare the body for sports practice instead of keeping a muscle stretched in a fixed position. Stretching becomes both a deactivation and activation on the same occasion, which benefits those who have an imminent achievement.

STATIC STRETCH

The practitioner stretches himself to fixed positions and a specific position is held with the muscle extended. Static stretching is exercised before and after a performance.

SCIENCE COMPARES STATIC AND DYNAMIC STRETCHING

The research results indicate that dynamic stretching can increase acute muscle power to a greater extent than static. These results can have important consequences for athletes participating in events that rely on high muscle power. Several researchers have compared static and dynamic stretching to strength and performance. Several studies have not found any improvement in performance when comparing static and dynamic stretching. Unlike static stretching, dynamic stretching is not associated with strength or performance failure.

The literature mixes the effects of stretching before exercise, as varming up. Some researchers report that static stretching after varming up reduces performance. Another study compared three heating protocols and the results indicated that dynamic stretching has greater utility in improving performance on power output compared to static stretching.

An interesting study was to show the influence of static and dynamic stretching in the upper body. In general, there was no short-term effect of stretching in the upper body of young adult male athletes, regardless of stretching mode. Because throwing performance was largely unaffected by static or dynamic upper body stretching, athletes who compete can perform upper body stretching.

There is significant evidence that static stretching can inhibit performance in strength and power activities. However, most of this research has involved stretching routines that differ from those practiced by athletes. This suggests that in practice a subsequent high-intensity warm-up restored the differences between the periods.

Researchers reported that after four repetitions, there was little change, which means that a minimum number of stretch repetitions lead to most of the extension in repetitive stretching. In addition, higher peak tension and energy absorption occurred at faster stretch rates, suggesting that the risk of injury in a stretching exercise may be related to speed and not to actual technology. The group of people who need stretching most is also susceptible and can be harmed by aggressive stretching.

Some injuries have been reported by stretching and some practitioners may seek out physiotherapists for rehabilitation. Of course, stretching can be practiced in an inaccurate manner – Stretch muscles not muscle tendons.

A systematic review of the literature was made to assess the effect of static stretching as part of warm-up, for prevention of exercise-related injuries. There is moderate to strong evidence that routine static stretching does not reduce overall injury risk. However, there is preliminary evidence that static stretching can reduce muscle damage.

Fitness program, for a general training program, recommends the American College of Sports Medicine static stretching:

- For most people before active warm-up
- At least 2 to 3 days per week
- Stretch for 15-30 seconds and repeat 2 to 4 times
- Older adults may need 60 seconds

Many training studies on older adults include stretch exercises as part of an exercise program. Older adults may need longer stretching times than the recommended 15 to 30 seconds. Researchers found that 60 seconds of static stretch holdings were associated with greater improvements in posterior thigh flexibility in older adults compared to shorter duration. The effectiveness of the type of stretching seems to be related to age and gender. Men and older adults under the age of 65 respond better to dynamic stretching. While women and older adults over 65 benefit from static stretching. These facts also suggest that muscle training decreases with age.

Static and dynamic stretching are all effective methods for increased flexibility and muscle relaxation, but several authors have noted an individualized response to stretching, therefore stretching programs need to be individualized.

This fact is in direct harmony with my own experience and points out that it would be the variation of muscle types and fitness status that more reflects the actual effectiveness of stretching.

The literature usually supports stretching to increase the individual's flexibility. Warm-up in sports and exercise is stretching as part of a pre-workout and is intended to reduce passive stiffness and increase movement during exercise. Generally, it appears that static stretching is most advantageous for athletes who require flexibility for their sports. Dynamic stretching can be better suited for athletes who need to run or jump as basketball players or sprinters.

The research is limited by the permanent effects of static stretching, however, muscle relaxation is greatest immediately after a stretch and a period of 15 minutes is usually a prevailing idea when the peak has been achieved. The important thing is that after a stretching exercise, bedding should not wait too long, because the relaxation and shifting of the nervous system is what is to be achieved.

RANGE OF MOMENT-ROM

The greatest change in ROM with static stretching occurs between 15 and 30 seconds and is sufficient to increase flexibility, according to most authors. In addition, no increase in muscle extension occurs after 4 repetitions. Static stretching has been shown to reduce muscle strength. The loss of strength derived from acute static stretching has been called "stretch-induced strength loss". The specific causes of this type of stretch-induced loss in strength are not clear; some suggest neural factors, while others mechanical factors.

Human movement is dependent on how much range of motion (ROM) is present in the synovial joint, like in the joint of elbow, hip and knee. In general, the movement can be limited to two anatomical units: joints and muscles. Muscles provide both passive and active tension:

- Passive muscle tension, depending on the structure of the muscle and surrounding facia.
- Active muscle tension.

Passive muscle tension is of the highest interest, as factors such as muscle structure and facia lead to the Type 1 muscle. Many of these fiber bundles provide another muscle construction in general.

RESTLESS LEG SYNDROME

This common syndrome is appropriate to describe further as surely many people have mild RLS is a common, under-diagnosed neurological movement disorder of a not fully understood etiology. Peripheral nerve abnormalities have been suggested, but no associated structural changes in the nerve end have been identified. The primary treatments for RLS are pharmacological and are a common neurological movement disorder that affects a large segment of the population. Most clinical trials have concentrated on the use of dopamine and benzodiazepines with multiple preparations, which often have significant side effects. Patients with RLS have a characteristic difficulty trying to describe their symptoms. They can report feelings as an almost irresistible desire to touch the legs, which are not painful but are clearly disturbing. This can lead to significant physical and emotional impairment. Sensations are usually inferior during inactivity, leading to discomfort, stress and insomnia. General effects are usually set at about 10-15% of the population, where men and women are equally affected, but are often misdiagnosed.

It is not too far-fetched to conclude that the inner calf muscle Soleus, among other factors, is at the top of this medical drama. With 65+% Type 1 fibers in the body, most of all skeletal muscles, there must be a connection. In case of mild ailment, stretching can be used advantageously for the moment to overcome the irritating cravings.

The symptoms are usually experienced worse in the evening and at night and usually ameliorated in the morning. One cause, in the morning all day hormones begin to be pumped into the body. The cortisol is like the highest in the morning, after 5:00. In more severe cases, symptoms may be present throughout the day with no circadian rhythm variation. Other features usually associated with RLS but not required for diagnosis include sleep disturbances and fatigue of the day. The symptoms usually progress slowly with an increasing disturbance of sleep. RLS symptoms occur in 25-50% of patients with iron deficiency. RLS is associated with reduced quality of life.

Epidemiological studies have shown a link between RLS and physical activity. A randomized controlled trial was designed to evaluate the effects of an exercise program on the symptoms of RLS. The improvement in RLS symptoms occurred as early as 6 weeks, which was similar to the time of regular pharmaceutical treatments and the decrease in RLS symptoms was maintained throughout the 3-month intervention period. No attempts were made in this study to distinguish between the effects of aerobic and resistance training. Future studies should evaluate the effectiveness of different types of exercise, the researchers concluded. RLS symptoms are favored by Type 1 fibers and in the short term, stretching is preferred relief, whereas resistance training should increase Typ2 fibers and eventually reduce RLS symptoms.

STRETCHING AND SLEEP FOR ADULTS

For most people, the sleep engine is weakened by age, as evidenced by many scientific reports. The reason for lower sleep capacity through aging is not fully understood and the scientific establishment has different conclusions on this subject. Many elderly people sleep on the margin and need a way to improve sleep quality, feel better and live a normal life. A muscle needs to be activated and that it is even more important during aging. It is surely a truth, that the deactivate/wasted muscles follow the same curves in the diagram as the lack of quality sleep. Activating some muscles and stretching others is a good habit of building up good sleep for everyone.

SUMMARY

Proprioceptors are found in all nerve endings in joints, muscles and tendons. The proprioceptors read the muscle's status in work as rest, which is of great importance for how the muscle tension affects a weak sleep engine.

***

Stretch for 15-30 seconds and repeat 2 to 4 times. Older adults may need 60 seconds. At least 2 to 3 days per week, but can be used advantageously before bedtime.

***

If you have a weak sleep engine and signals that correspond to muscle tension, it is more difficult to achieve Alfarytm, the precursor of sleep.

***

Passive muscle tension is of the highest interest, as factors such as muscle structure and facia lead to the Type 1 muscle. Many of these fiber bundles provide another muscle construction in general.

***

The greatest change in ROM with static stretching occurs between 15 and 30 seconds and is sufficient to increase flexibility, according to most authors.

***

The inner calf muscle with 65+% Type 1 fibers, most of all skeletal muscles, can be used advantageously by stretching to get over the annoying creeps at the moment.

***

Deactivating before bedtime

For a person with a weak sleep engine, sleep will not come naturally. Practicing stretching means, that you get more benefits than just improving sleep quality. The bone motor has an influence on the bowel movement has been clear for a long time, but relaxed leg muscles also have a greater impact on the bowel movement. The gastrointestinal tract becomes relaxed during regular stretching as bowel obstruction blocks the body's relaxation ability. The abdominal region has a great influence on the ability to relax at bedtime.

Exercising several times, a week and building muscle will improve your sleep skills, but for predominantly Type1 fibers, stretching is needed as a deactivation. This method is easy to learn for almost everyone, training and stretching is something that many have already tried. The legs represent the perfect symbiosis for the activation / deactivation methodology when the thighs stand for strength and the calves for endurance. Stretching is for the moment and should be exercised immediately for bedtime.

Make this a good habit every night before you go to bed. It only takes ten minutes, but it will be the best invested minutes in your life.

DEACTIVATING 1 – FRONT OF THIGH

The thigh muscle is one of the larger muscles in the body that supports movement and transport. It generally requires more exercise time than other muscles to become relaxed.

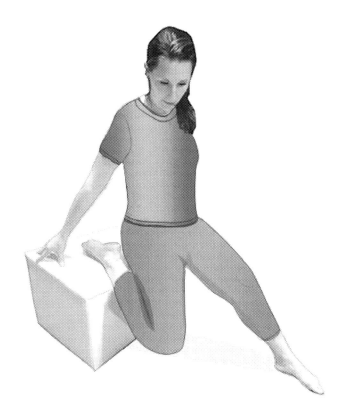

Figure 14. Front of thigh

Front thighs provide the most relaxation after stretching, in my experience. It is a large, strong muscle group, but takes it easy in the beginning.

Important! Do not do this exercise if you have an unstable or operated knee joint. Or ask a doctor.

IMPLEMENTATION

Stretch the thigh by placing the foot on a soft surface. Bend your thigh down while stretching your back. Tipping the back a little backwards, or for the thigh down, feels a clear stretch in the front thigh. Remember not to strain your ankle. It is important to use a soft surface, such as a sofa or a bed. Try to keep this position for a while. Important exercise for the end result; relaxation.

Stretching time depends a lot on the current stress level and muscle tone. This first stretch exercise is most important because of the size and strength of the muscle. Give the exercise time to feel the relaxation. Already, the stress level may have fallen and thus the first yawning can come as on order.

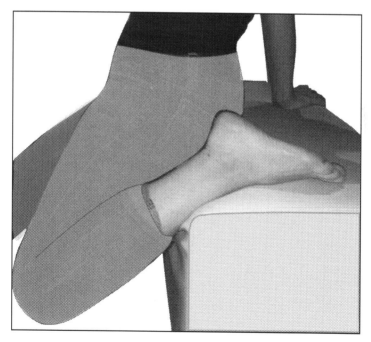

Figure 15. Thigh stretch, detail

Important!

Place the foot on a soft surface. Use a pillow or fold a towel under the foot if the substrate is hard.

The foot and lower leg should form an angle so that the pressure is felt on the thigh and not in the ankle. Also, keep in mind if possible, have as little angle as possible between the thigh and the lower leg.

NOTE! This stretch can be done in different ways, sitting, standing or lying down, by lifting the foot with muscle force against the seat. The most convenient and practical is to sit to use your own body weight as a counterweight. With a little exercise, both thighs can be stretched simultaneously to shorten the time. But in that case a very soft surface is required and the exercise is not recommended at first.

DEACTIVATING 2 – OUTER CALF

The calf has most TYP-1 fibers among the body's skeletal muscles and therefore important to stretch. The first part of the program describes the essential stretching exercises; stretch of lower body and legs. Remember that the relaxation effect can shift from muscle to muscle and also vary between different stretching occasions.

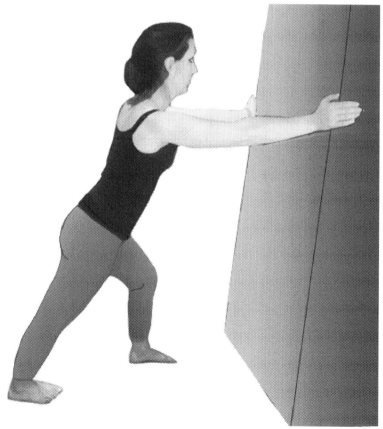

Figure 16. Outer calf stretch

When practicing the stretching program you get a better overall health as many blockages in the abdominal region release. Stretch your calf muscles before continuing with the back thighs. The calf muscles are not the largest muscles but are strong and adapted to work for a long time. The status of the calf muscles is of great importance to your well-being.

IMPLEMENTATION

Place your hands against a wall and lean your body against it. The stretching pad is placed behind the vertical of the upper body. The angle of the leg determines the stretching of the calf and more inclination of the body towards the wall provides more stretching. The stretch is felt throughout the leg, but especially in M. Gastrocnemius.

DEACTIVATING 3 – BACK OF THIGH

The program continues with the back thigh or hoarding. This muscle pack is also strong which requires some work to get relaxed. My experience and feeling is that the muscle does not have the same elasticity, more dumb/stiff compared to the front thigh.

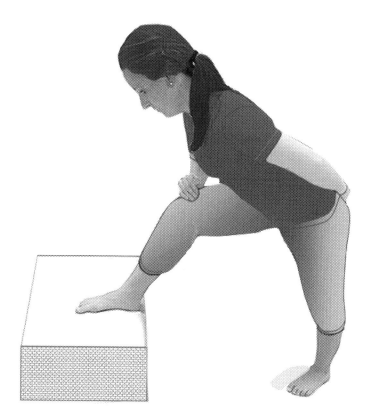

Figure 17. Back of thigh stretch

You have already got a good relaxation after calf stretch, but remember that stretching can affect more muscles than just those indicated by the exercises.

IMPLEMENTATION

Place the stretching leg on a sofa or pallet. The thigh and lower leg should form a 45 degree angle. Tilt over to the thigh. The angle now makes the entire stretch feel only in the thigh. The muscles are strong here, so be patient. Tilt over and relax.

DEACTIVATING 4 – BACK OF LEG

To provide additional relaxation, a combination exercise fol-lows. This is a final exercise for the entire back of the thigh and should be facilitated by what has already been done before. Take it easy, as it can tighten one part on the back of the knee.

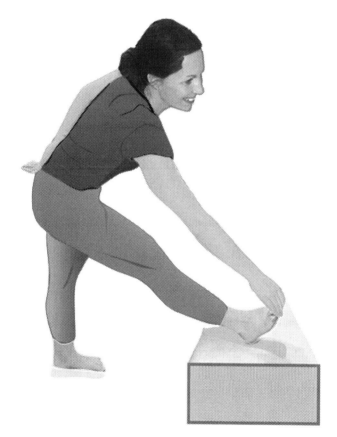

Figure 18. Back of leg stretch

Normally, this exercise is practiced with a straight leg. Stand up, place the stretching leg on a chair or the like, bend the upper body forward and grasp the toes.

DEACTIVATING 5 - GLUTEUS
Maximus, Medius, Minimus

Continue with the last exercise in this first stretch part. It is an important exercise for sleep and for your hips. The muscle group consists of three muscles that work under different leg angles.

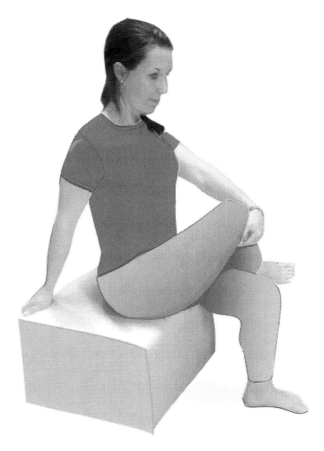

Figure 19. Gluteus muscles stretch

IMPLEMENTATION

Sit on the bed edge and grasp the foot on the side you intend to stretch. Put the leg on top of the opposite thigh and pull the leg towards you. Pull with both arms and press the leg against the body. Only a minor stabilizing force is used through the foot so as not to compromise the knee joint. This exercise can also be done lying down.

M. Gluteus consists of three muscles. When the leg is pulled toward the center of the torso, the maximus is stretched. When the leg is pulled more towards the same side, medius and minimus are stretched.

Because of the angle, different muscles are activated. Variation and practice gives information what feels best.

Take it easy if you have any problems with your hips. Some pain may occur due to tense M. Gluteus. They can feel tense and hard. Use a soft but firm movement.

PART 2
DEACTIVATING 6 – NECK

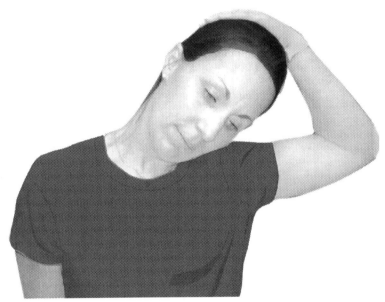

Figure 20. Neck stretch

IMPLEMENTATION

You can stand or sit while doing this exercise, Fix the shoulder that otherwise accompanies the movement and then the stroke is not correct. To remedy and stabilize the shaft take a firm grip in any solid object or chair. Grab your head with the opposite hand / arm of the side. Tighten the side with a smooth movement.

Pain in the neck muscles is common and it can give a good response to stretching these muscles. There is a bunch of muscles in this area and it is no great idea to distinguish them. M. Trapezius is the largest and may be the target muscle.

DEACTIVATION 7 - NECK, UPPER

This part of the neck can quickly become sore and stiff during stressful periods.

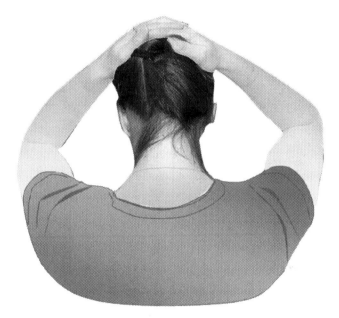

Figure 21. Upper neck stretch

Common with pain around the shell base, as the area consisting of a number of small muscles helps the head to be fixed at the neck. These are also fixed at the first neck vertebra, also called the atlas car.

IMPLEMENTATION

Grasp the head firmly with both hands at the same time. Gently pull your head forward toward your chest with a gentle and slow motion. Then a reverse movement is made. Bend back your head, just with the weight / force of your hands and arms, no extra weight. Repeat the movement.

AVACTIVATION 8 - SHOULDER

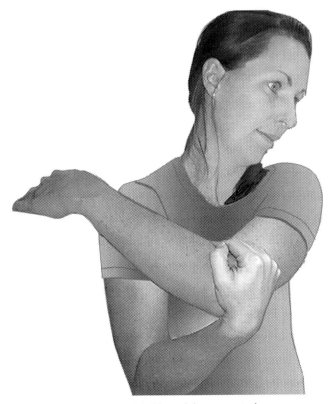

Figure 22. Shoulder stretch

IMPLEMENTATION

Sit or stand. Hold the stretching arm at ninety degrees from the body and at the same angle in the elbow. Take a firm grip around your elbow with your other hand and pull the other side.

DEACTIVATION 9 — LOWER ARM

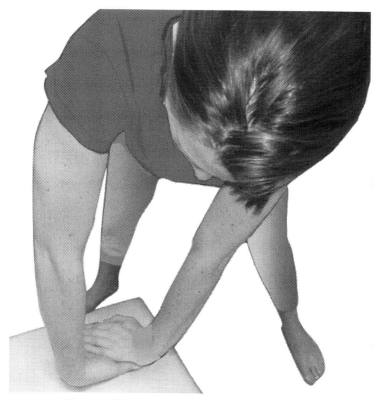

Figure 23 Front of lower arm stretch

IMPLEMENTATION

Preferably use a soft surface. These muscles are small and easy to work with. Place your hand on the surface; bend the outside of the hand against the surface. The fingers can point to the body or turn the arm ninety degrees outwards, making the stroke more effective.

FAST GUIDE PART -1A

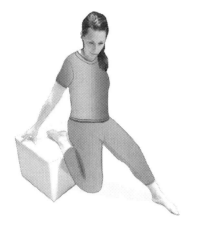

Deactivating 1
Front of thigh
Stretch time: 2 minutes

Important stretch for the end resultat.

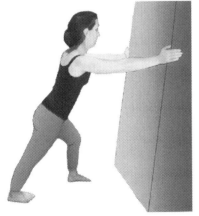

Deactivating 2
Calf
Stretch time: 1 minut

Good stretch if you have "creepy feeling" in legs; can alleviate a lot.

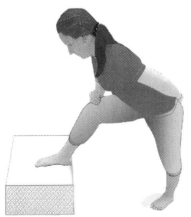

Deactivating 3
Back of thigh
Stretch time: 1 min

Tight and hard muscles. For full effect; lean forward with straight back and chest towards of the thigh.

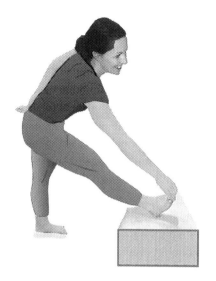

Back o f leg
Stretch time: 0,5 - 1 minut

A stretch that combines calf and back thigh stretch.

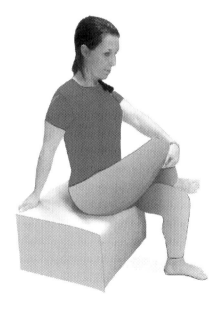

Deactivating 5 Gluteus
Stretch time: 0,5 - 1 minut

Remember to angle the power direction to activate all Gluteus muscles; mini, media and maximus.

FAST GUIDE PART -1B

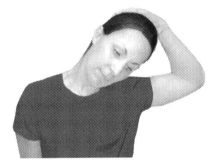

**Deactivating 6
Neck
Stretch time: 0.5 minut**

Easy to experience pain.

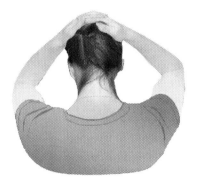

**Deactivating 7
Neck bow
Stretch time: 0.5 min**

The neck bow's muscles are among the first muscles to lock in stress.

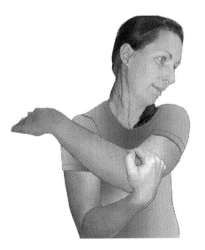

**Deactivating 8
Choulder
Stretch tim: 0.5 min**

Easy to stretch.

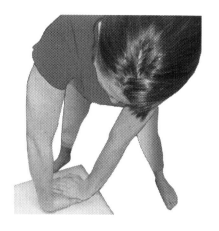

Deactivating 9
Front of lower arm
Stretch time: 0.5 minut

Good stretch for computer work, sleep and for preventing tennis elbow.

PART 2 - ACTIVATION

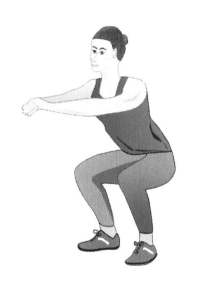

Activating 1 - Squats
Thigh and gluteus
Activation time: 30-60 sek

A brief activation to give the body the right impulses and to balance stretching.

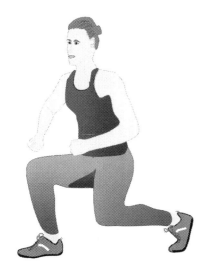

Activating 1b Stationary Outcome / Leg
Activating time: 30-60 sek

An alternative to the first exercise. Short stitch length, 10 cm, to activate muscles the most.

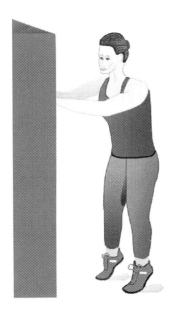

Activation 2 Toe press / Calf
Aktivation time: 30-60 sek

Good exercise to pump the calves, to give a good result on sleep skills.

Implication

A variety of research reports show the importance of the muscles for the individual's well-being. Much has been written about the muscles and condition of the cardiovascular system and the brain with several areas. Many researchers now also report the importance of muscles for the quality of sleep, even at high age. This book describes how activation of the strong muscles can be balanced with deactivation of the weak.

Fewer movements make the human body more susceptible to anxiety and stress. Many studies support relaxation exercise to reduce stress and thus relaxation training becomes an increasingly common form of treatment.

People suffering from insomnia show significantly reduced BDNF levels in blood serum. Physical exercise increase circulating BDNF levels. A single exercise exercise increases the amount of subsequent SWS, slow sleep waves. Type 2 muscle fibers are increased in strength-training individuals, which reduce the loss of muscle mass.

MISCONCEPTION

During my time with stretch relaxation courss, there has sometimes been a clear idea among participants, that one cannot stretch without warm-up, an idea which must, however, be taken seriously. The science shows that stretching can be exercised both before and after a workout. My feeling has been that this notion applies only to the legs. No one would have an idea of stretching a stiff neck. However, stiff bones need deactivation. With the new activation supplement before bedtime use, that can be used before stretching, this dilemma resolves.

I have never had any negative experience during all years of stretching and with muscle activation that has developed over the last few years, I now hope to reach a wider crowd of people in need. For everyone it is unique and can therefore need an arsenal of tools to improve sleep. Some people do not need stretching, those with fewer numbers of slow muscles. They probably need activation of the strong muscles. Even if you are born with Type 2 fibers, they are not strong throughout life - volume before strength. The importance of the legs for sleep cannot be overestimated, they are important. The legs have the largest muscles in the body and even the weakest, they are a balance pool for a safe sleep status.

Keep in mind that the legs have the two muscle types in quantities, but they are in different places. This is the basis for:

MUSCLE / SLEEP METHODOLOGY

- Calf, Typ 1-fibre=deactivation
- Thigh, Typ 2-fibre=activation

The exercises have been developed and adapted to today's modern man. Over time, many users will surely develop and adapt the method for themselves, which will only make the exercises even more effective. In addition, this method can be combined with any other therapy. The most important thing is to be careful about the time aspect and to wait for answers from the body. Deactivation and activation are for the moment. The right time is important, there is a "peak moment" as it is especially important to go to bed. Allow deactivation and activation to do their job.

However, building muscle is best done in the gym. To have strong legs make all movements easy, as well as getting better quality sleep. The activation before bedtime is only a short while and does not make sense to raise the body temperature significantly. When exercising the program, the body will emit signs of response, such as yawning and gurgling, vibrating sounds. These signs are due to blockages, mainly in the abdominal region being dissolved and a sign that a change of nervous system has begun. The alert system is being broken down to the benefit of the night system. Take advantage of this fact - GO TO BED!

GOOD LUCK!

References

INTRODUCTION

Sundelin T, Lekander M, Kecklund G, Van Someren EJ, Olsson A, Axelsson J; Cues of fatigue: effects of sleep deprivation on facial appearance; Sleep. 2013 Sep 1; 36(9):1355-60. Doi: 10.5665/ sleep.2964.

http://www.unt.se/uppland/uppsala/somnen-skyddar-hjarnan-2680489.aspx, Källa: http://www.journalsleep.org/Accepted Papers/SP-100-13.pdf

Benzodiazepine use and risk of Alzheimer's disease: case-control studyBMJ 2014; 349 doi: https://doi.org/10.1136/bmj.g5205 (Published 09 September 2014) Cite this as: BMJ 2014; 349: g5205

Jane E. Ferrie, Meena Kumari, Paula Salo, Archana Singh-Manoux, Mika Kivimäki; Sleep epidemiology—a rapidly growing field; Int J Epidemiol. Author manuscript: available in PMC. 2013. May 17; Int. J. Epidemiol. 2011 Dec; 40(6): 1431–1437.doi: 10.1093/ije/dyr203. PMCID: PMC3655374. HALMS: HALMS677212. PMID: 22158659

Gallicchio L, Kalesan B; Sleep duration and mortality: a systematic review and meta-analysis; Sleep Res. 2009 Jun; 18 (2): 148-58. Doi: 10.1111/j.1365-2869.2008.00732.x.

WHO; Electromagnetic fields and public health; June 2007 http://www.who.int/peh-emf/publications/facts/fs322/en/

https://www.folkhalsomyndigheten.se/livsvillkor-levnadsvanor/ miljohalsa-och-halsoskydd/inomhusmiljo-allmanna-lokaler-och-platser/elektromagnetiska-falt/

Lennart Hardell, Michael Carlberg; Mobile phone and cordless phone use and the risk for glioma – Analysis of pooled case-control studies in Sweden, 1997–2003 and 2007–2009;

Pathophysiology, Volume 22, Issue 1, March 2015, Pages 1-13 https://doi.org/10.1016/j.pathophys.2014.10.001

http://www.stralskyddsstiftelsen.se/wp-content/uploads/2014/08/risk_tumor_huvud_201406.pdf

http://www.riksdagen.se/sv/dokument-lagar/dokument/motion/eloverkanslighet_GY02F%C3%B6249

STRESS

Sheps D S; Mental stress may hurt the heart; University of Florida, posted in Journal of the American College of Cardiology.

G M Manzoni, F Pagnini, G Castelnuovo, E Molinari; Relaxation training for anxiety: a Ten-year systematic review with meta-analysis; BMC Psychiatry20088:41. Https: //doi. org/ 10.1186/ 1471-244X-8-41; Manzoni et al; licensee BioMed Central Ltd. 2008.

REF1. Somers JM, Goldner EM, Waraich P, Hsu L; Prevalence and incidence studies of anxiety disorders: a systematic review of the literature; Can J Psychiatry. 2006 Feb; 51(2):100-13.

REF15. Esch T, Fricchione GL, Stefano GB. The therapeutic use of the relaxation response in stress-related diseases. Med. Sci. Monit. 2003 Feb; 9 (2):RA23-34.

Lampert R, Tuit K, Hong KI, Donovan T, Lee F, Sinha R; Cumulative stress and autonomic dysregulation in a community sample; Stress (Amsterdam, Netherlands). 2016 Apr 25; 19(3): 269-279. Doi: 10.1080/10253890.2016. 1174847.

Matthew A. Stults-Kolehmainen, Keri Tuit, Rajita Sinha; Lower cumulative stress is associated with better health for physically active adults in the community; Stress. 2014 Mar; 17(2): 157–168. Published online 2014 Jan 29. Doi: 10.3109/10253890. 2013.878329. PMCID: PMC4548889. NIHMSID: NIHMS708772

McEwen BS, Gianaros PJ. Central role of the brain in stress and adaptation: links to socioeconomic status, health, and disease; Annals of the New York Academy of Sciences 2010.

ADRENAL FATIGUE

Dement W C and Vaughan C; the promise of sleep: a pioneer in sleep medicine explores the vital connection between health, happiness, and a good night's sleep; New York: Delacorte Press. 1999

http://ww2.lakartidningen.se/store/articlepdf/1/16560/1196_1198.pdf

http://halsantillbaka.nu/binjurar/

Penev P; when dieting to lose weight, how much you sleep may be as important as how much you eat; publ. in

Annals of Internal Medicine; the Journal of the America College of Physicians

Glenn AL, Raine A, Schug RA, GAO Y. Granger DA; Increased testosterone to cortisol ratio in psychopathy; J. Abnorm Psychol. 2011; 120: 389–399.

Linton S J; Does work stress predict insomnia? A prospective study. Br J Health Psychol. 2004. 9: 127–136.

Dr. Ingaramo, MD, vid American Society of Hypertension. Psykisk stress kan således associeras med organskador.

INSOMNIA

Sadeka Tamanna, Stephen A. Geraci; Major sleep disorders among women; South Med J. 2013; 106(8):470-478.

Insomnia in the Young May Have Genetic Basis
David Douglas, Reuters Health Information, January 13, 2015

Senior author Michael Grandner; SLEEP 2018: 32nd Annual Meeting of the Associated Professional Sleep Societies. Abstract0189. Presented June 4. 2018.

Mario Giovanni Terzano; Liborio Parrino; Enrica Bonanni; Fabio Cirignotta; Franco Ferrillo; Gian Luigi Gigli; Mariantonietta Savarese; Luigi Ferini-Strambi; Insomnia in General Practice; A Consensus Report Produced by Sleep Specialists and Primary-Care Physicians in Italy; Posted 12/22/2005

Mona Mohamed, Ibrahim Abdalla. Ghrelin–Physiological functions and regulation; Eur. Endocrinol. 2015 Aug; 11(2): 90–95. Published online 2015 Aug 19. Doi:

10.17925/ EE.2015. 11.02.90 PMCID: PMC5819073, PMID: 29632576

CIRKADIAN RHYTHM

Horne JA, Östberg O (1976). A self-assessment questionnaire to determine morningness-eveningness in human circadian rhythms. Int J Chronobiol 4 (2): Sid. 97–110. PMID 1027738.

Brianna D. Harfmann, Elizabeth A. Schroder, Karyn A. Esser. Circadian rhythms, the molecular clock, and Skeletal Muscl; J Biol Rhythms. 2015 Apr; 30(2): 84–94; Published online 2014 Dec 15. doi: 10.1177/ 0748730414561638. PMCID: PMC447 0613. NIHMSID: NIHMS696340

https://www.researchgate.net/publication/51416434_Role_ of_MyoD_in_denervated_disused_and_exercised_ muscle

Chatterjee S, Nam D, Guo B, Kim JM, Winnier GE, Lee J, Berdeaux R, Yechoor VK, Ma K. Brain and muscle Arnt-like 1 is a key regulator of myogenesis; Journal of cell science. 2013; 126: 2213–2224.

Bass J, Takahashi J S; Circadian integration of metabolism and energetics. 2010. Science 330, 1349–1354 10.1126/ science. 1195027

Dubrovsky YV, Samsa WE, Kondratov RV; Deficiency of circadian protein CLOCK reduces lifespan and increases age-related cataract development in mice. Aging. 2010;2:936–944.

Kondratov R. V., Kondratova A. A., Gorbacheva V. Y., Vykhovanets O. V., Antoch M. P. (2006). Early aging and age-related pathologies in mice deficient in BMAL1, the core componentof the circadian clock; Genes Dev. 20, 1868–1873 10.1101/gad.1432206

Dyar KA, Ciciliot S, Wright LE, Bienso RS, Tagliazucchi GM, Patel VR, Forcato M, Paz MI, Gudiksen A, Solagna F, et al. Muscle insulin sensitivity and glucose metabolism are controlled by the intrinsic muscle clock. Mol. Metab. 2014. 3: 29–41.

Buhr ED, Takahashi JS; Molecular components of the mammalian circadian clock. Handb Exp Pharmacol. 2013; 217:3–27

O'Neill JS, Reddy AB. Circadian clocks in human red blood cells. Nature. 2011. 469: 498–503.

Andrews J. L., Zhang X., McCarthy J. J., McDearmon E. L., Hornberger T. A., Russell B., Campbell K. S., Arbogast S., Reid M. B., Walker J. R. et al. (2010). CLOCK and BMAL1 regulate MyoD and are necessary for maintenance of skeletal muscle phenotype and function. Proc. Natl. Acad. Sci. USA 107, 19090–19095 10,1073/pnas.1014523107

Wolff G, Esser KA. Scheduled exercise phase shifts the circadian clock in skeletal muscle. Med Sci Sports Exerc. 2012; 44:1663–1670.

Wilson J; the 21st Century stress syndrome; Publ. by Smart Publications Petaluma,

Loomis A L, Harvey E N, Hobart G A. Cerebral states during sleep as studies by human brain potentials. J Exp Psychol 1937; 21:127–44

Lowry F; Insufficient Sleep Thwarts Weight Loss Efforts; Medscape Medical News

MUSCLES AND SLEEP IN SPACE

Cotter Joshua A; Yu Alvin; Haddad Fadia; Kreitenberg Arthur; Baker Michael J; Tesch Per A; Baldwin Kenneth M; Caiozzo Vincent J; Adams Gregory R; Concurrent Exercise on a Gravity-independent Device During Simulated Microgravity; Med Sci Sports Exerc. 2015; 47(5):990-1000

Graeber R C 1, Rosekind M R 1, Connell L J 1 and Dinges D F 2; 1. Cockpit Napping Flight Human Factors Branch; NSA Ames Research Center 2 Institute of Pennsylvania Hospital; University of Pennsylvania School of Medicine

Patrick L. Barry, Dr. Tony Phillips; NASA Naps; Science@NASA https://www.nasa.gov/vision/space/livinginspace/03jun_naps.html

Monk TH, Monk TH, Hobson JA, Moldofsky H, Ponomareva I, Principal Investigators; Sleep Investigations http://spaceflight. nasa.gov/ history/shuttle-mir/science/hls/neuro/sc-hls-sleep.htm

Rosemary Wilson; Wide Awake in Outer Space; Science@NASA. https://www.nasa.gov/audience/forstudents/5-8/features/ to_sleep feature.html

MYOCINES

Erickson KI, Voss MW, Prakash RS, Basak C, Szabo A, Chaddock L, et al. Exercise training increases size of hippocampus and improves memory. Proc Natl Acad Sci U S A. 2011; 108(7):3017–22. http://dx.doi.org/10.1073/pnas.1015950108. ; PubMed Central PMCID: PMCPMC3041121. Doi: 10.1073/pnas.1015950108

Byunghun So, Hee-Jae Kim, Jinsoo Kim, and Wook Song; Exercise-induced myokines in health and metabolic diseases; Integr Med Res. 2014 Dec; 3(4): 172–179. Published online 2014 Oct 5. Doi: 10.1016/j.imr.2014.09.007. PMCID: PMC5481763

https://www.psychologytoday.com/us/blog/the-athletes-way/201610/irisin-the-exercise-hormone-is-fat-fighting-phenomenon

Nielsen AR, Pedersen BK. The biological roles of exercise-induced cytokines: IL-6, IL-8, and IL-15. Appl Physiol Nutr Metab. 2007; 32: 833–839.

Costanzo, Linda S. (2002). Physiology (2nd ed.). Philadelphia: Saunders. p. 23. ISBN 0-7216-9549-3.

McGuff, Doug, MD. The Amazing Power of Myokines. http://www.bodybyscience.net/home.html/?p=1340 12 January 2014.

Rawson ES, Venezia AC; Use of creatine in the elderly and evidence for effects on cognitive function in young and old; Amino Acids. 2011 May; 40(5):1349-62. Doi: 10.1007/s00726-011-0855-9. Epub 2011 Mar 11.

BDNF-SLEEP MYOCINES HOLY GRAIL

Kirk I. Erickson; Exercise training increases size of hippocampus and improves memory." The Proceedings of the National Academy of Sciences vol. 108 no. 7 > 3017–3022, doi: 10.1073/pnas.1015950108

Eric J Huang, Louis F Reichardt; Neurotrophins: Roles in Neuronal Development and Function; Annu Rev Neurosci. Author manuscript; available in PMC 2009, Oct 6. Published in final edited form as: Annu Rev

Neurosci. 2001; 24: 677–736. Doi: 10.1146/ annurev. neuro.24.1 .677. PMCID: PMC2758233; NIHMSID: NIHMS112782, PMID: 11520916.

Jonato Prestes, Dahan da Cunha Nascimento, Ramires Alsamir Tibana, Tatiane Gomes Teixeira,Denis Cesar Leite Vieira, Vitor Tajra, Darlan Lopes de Farias, Alessandro Oliveira Silva, Silvana Schwerz Funghetto,Vinicius Carolino de Souza, and James Wilfred Navalta; Understanding the individual responsiveness to resistance training periodization; Age (Dordr). 2015 Jun; 37(3): 55. Published online 2015 May 14. doi: 10.1007/s11357-015-9793-x-PMCID: PMC4430497PMID: 25971877

MariaGiese, EvaUnternaehrer, SergeBrand, PasqualeCalabrese, Edith Holsboer-Trachsler, Anne Eckert, Kenji Hashimoto, Edito; The Interplay of Stress and Sleep Impacts BDNF Level; PLoS One. 2013; 8(10): e76050. Published online 2013 Oct 16. Doi: 10.1371/ journal.pone.0076050 PMCID: PMC3797810 PMID: 24146812

Karege F, Perret G, Bondolfi G, Schwald M, Bertschy G, et al. (2002) Decreased serum brain-derived neurotrophic factor levels in major depressed patients. Psychiatry Res 109: 143–148. [PubMed]

M Giese, E Unternährer, H Hüttig, J Beck, S Brand, P Calabrese, E Holsboer-Trachsler, A Eckert; BDNF: an indicator of insomnia? Mol. Psychiatry. 2014 Feb; 19(2): 151–152. Published online 2013 Feb 12. Doi: 10.1038/ mp. 2013.10. PMCID: PMC3903111.

B. Rael Cahn, Matthew S. Goodman, Christine T. Peterson, Raj Maturi, Paul J. Mills; Awakening response, and altered inflammatory marker expression after a 3-month yoga and meditation retreat; Front Hum Neurosci; 2017.

11,315. Published online 2017 Jun 26. Doi: 10.3389/fnhum.2017.00315
PMCID: PMC5483482, PMID: 28694775.

https://anatomifysiologi.se/fysiologi/nervsystemet/reflex/

Kanzleiter T, Rath M, Görgens SW, Jensen J, Tangen DS, Kolnes AJ, Kolnes KJ, Lee S, Eckel J, Schürmann A, and Eckardt K. "The myokine decorin is regulated by contraction and involved in muscle hypertrophy." Biochem Biophys Res Commun. 2014 Jul 1. Pii: S0006-291X (14)01197-8. Doi: 10.1016/j. bbrc.2014 .06.123.

Karan S. Rana, Muhammad Arif, Eric J. Hill, Sarah Aldred, David A. Nagel, Alan Neville, Harpal S. Randeva, Clifford J. Bailey, Srikanth Bellary & James E. Brown. "Plasma irisin levels predict telomere length in healthy adults." AGE (2014) 36:995–1001. DOI 10.1007/s11357-014-9620-9. Published online: 29 January 2014.

Timmons JA, Baar K, Davidsen PK, Atherton PJ (2012). "Is irisin a human exercise gene?" Nature 488 (7413): E9–10; discussion E10–1. Doi: 10.1038/nature11364. PMID 22932392

Boström P, Wu J, Jedrychowski MP, Korde A, Ye L, Lo JC, Rasbach KA, Boström EA, Choi JH, Long JZ, Kajimura S, Zingaretti MC, Vind BF, Tu H, Cinti S, Højlund K, Gygi SP, Spiegelman BM; A PGC1-α-dependent myokine that drives brown-fat-like development of white fat and thermogenesis; Nature. 2012 Jan 11; 481(7382):463-8. Doi: 10.1038/nature10777.

Peng Zheng, Xiaohong Xu, Hongyan Zhao, Tingting Lv, Bailin Song, 2 and Fuchun Wang; Tranquilizing and Allaying Excitement Needling Method Affects BDNF and SYP Expression in Hippocampus; Evid Based Complement

Alternat Med. 2017; 2017: 8215949; Published online 2017 Jul6. Doi: 10.1155/ 2017/8215949

Schmitt K, Holsboer-Trachsler E, Eckert A; BDNF in sleep, insomnia, and sleep deprivation; Ann Med. 2016;48(1-2):42-51. Doi: 10.3109/07853890. 2015.1131327. Epub 2016 Jan 13.

Siresha Bathina, Undurti N. Das1Bio-Science Research Center, Gayatri Vidya Parishad College of Engineering, Visakhapatnam, India; Brain-derived neurotrophic factor and its clinical implications; Arch Med Sci. 2015 Dec 10; 11(6): 1164–1178. Published online 2015 Dec 11. Doi: 10.5114/aoms.2015.56342 PMCID: PMC4697050.

Pedersen BK, Pedersen M, Krabbe KS, Bruunsgaard H, Matthews VB, Febbraio MA; Role of exercise-induced brain-derived neurotrophic factor production in the regulation of energy homeostasis in mammals; Exp Physiol. 2009 Dec;94(12):1153-60. Doi: 10.1113/ expphysiol.2009.048561. Epub 2009 Sep 11.

Adam Dinoff, Nathan Herrmann, Walter Swardfager, Celina S. Liu, Chelsea Sherman, Sarah Chan, and Krista L. Lanctôt; The Effect of Exercise Training on Resting Concentrations of Peripheral Brain-Derived Neurotrophic Factor (BDNF): A Meta-Analysis; Published online 2016 Sep 22. Doi: 10.1371/journal. Pone.0163037. PMCID: PMC5033477.

Greenberg ME, Xu B, Lu B, Hempstead BL; New insights in the biology of BDNF synthesis and release: implications in CNS function. The Journal of neuroscience: the official journal of the Society for Neuroscience. 2009; 29(41):12764–7. Doi: 10.1523/JNEUROSCI.3566-09.2009. PMCID: PMCPMC3091387.

Schiffer T, Schulte S, Hollmann W, Bloch W, Struder HK; Effects of strength and endurance training on brain-derived neurotrophic factor and insulin-like growth factor 1 in humans; Horm Metab Res. 2009; 41(3):250–4. http://dx.doi.org/10.1055/s-0028-1093322. Doi: 10,1055/s-0028-109 33 22

Seifert T, Brassard P, Wissenberg M, Rasmussen P, Nordby P, Stallknecht B, et al. Endurance training enhances BDNF release from the human brain. Am J Physiol Regul Integr Comp Physiol. 2010; 298(2):R372–7. http://dx.doi.org/10.1152/ajpregu.00525. 2009. Doi: 10.1152/ajpregu.00525.2009

Yarrow JF, White LJ, McCoy SC, Borst SE. Training augments resistance exercise induced elevation of circulating brain derived neurotrophic factor (BDNF). Neurosci Lett. 2010;479(2):161–5. http://dx.doi.org/ 10,1016 /j. neulet.2010. 05 058. doi: 10,1016 /j.neulet.2 010,05.058

Klein AB, Williamson R, Santini MA, Clemmensen C, Ettrup A, Rios M, et al. Blood BDNF concentrations reflect brain-tissue BDNF levels across species. Int J Neuropsychopharmacol. 2011; 14(3):347–53. Doi: 10.1017/ S1461145710000738 .

Faraguna Ugo, Vyazovskiy Vladyslav V, Nelson Aaron B, Tononi Giulio, Cirelli Chiara; A CAUSAL ROLE FOR BDNF IN THE HOMEOSTATIC REGULATION OF SLEEP; J Neurosci. Author manuscript; available in PMC 2008 Dec 8.Published in final edited form as:J Neurosci. 2008 Apr 9; 28(15): 4088–4095. Doi: 10.1523/ JNEUROSCI.5510-07.2008. PMCID: PMC 2597531

Sunao Uchida, Kohei Shioda, Yuko Morita, Chie Kubota, Masashi Ganeko, Noriko Takeda; Exercise Effects on Sleep Physiology; Front Neurol. 2012; 3: 48. Published

online 2012 Apr 2. Doi: 10.3389/fneur.2012.00048.
PMCID: PMC3317043.
PMID: 22485106

UNTRAINED OR AGED MUSCLES

Kelaiditi E, Jennings A, Steves CJ, Skinner J, Cassidy A, MacGregor AJ, Welch AA; Measurements of skeletal muscle mass and power are positively related to a Mediterranean dietary pattern in women; Osteoporos Int. 2016 Nov;27(11):3251-3260.

Wilkerson GB, Bullard JT, Bartal DW; Identification of cardiometabolic risks among collegiate football players; Journal of athletic training. 2010; 45(1):67–74.

Newman AB, Kupelian V, Visser M, Simonsick EM, Goodpaster BH, Kritchevsky SB, Tylavsky FA, Rubin SM, Harris TB; Strength, but not muscle mass, is associated with mortality in the health, aging and body composition study cohort; J Gerontol A Biol Sci Med Sci. 2006 Jan;61(1):72-7.

Storer TW, Basaria S, Traustadottir T, Harman SM, Pencina K, Li Z, Travison TG, Miciek R, Tsitouras P, Hally K, Huang G, Bhasin S; Effects of Testosterone Supplementation for 3-Years on Muscle Performance and Physical Function in Older Men; J Clin Endocrinol Metab. 2016 Oct 18: jc20162771.

Küüsmaa M, Schumann M, Sedliak M, Kraemer WJ, Newton RU, Malinen JP, Nyman K, Häkkinen A, Häkkinen K; Effects of morning versus evening combined strength and endurance training on physical performance, muscle hypertrophy, and serum hormone concentrations; Appl Physiol Nutr Metab. 2016 Dec; 41(12):1285-1294.

Orsatti FL, Nunes PR, Souza AP, Martins FM, de Oliveira AA, Nomelini RS, Michelin MA, Murta EF; Predicting Functional Capacity from Measures of Muscle Mass in Postmenopausal Women; PM R. 2016 Oct 8. Pii: S1934-1482(16)30988-1. Doi: 10.1016/j.pmrj.2016.10.001.

Marques EA, Figueiredo P, Harris TB, Wanderley FA, Carvalho J; Are resistance and aerobic exercise training equally effective at improving knee muscle strength and balance in older women? Arch Gerontol Geriatr. 2016 Oct. 11; 68: 106 - 112. Doi: 10.1016/ j.archger.2016.10.002.

Yvonne L. Eaglehouse, Evelyn O. Talbott, Yuefang Chang, Lewis H. Kuller; Participation in Physical Activity and Risk for Amyotrophic Lateral Sclerosis Mortality Among Postmenopausal Women; JAMA Neurol. 2016;73(3):329-336.doi:10.1001/ jamaneurol.2015.4487

Gligoroska JP, Manchevska S; The effects of physical activities on cognition—physiological mechanism; Mater. 2012; 24(3):198–202. http://dx.doi.org/ 10.5455/ msm.2012.24.198-202. ; PubMed Central PMCID: PMCPMC3633396.

http://coachmikeblogs.com/chronic-cardio-aging-muscle-fibers/ #sthash. IHTjrHOw.dpuf

Robert H. Fitts, James R. Peters, E. Lichar Dillon, William J. Durham, Melinda Sheffield-Moore, and Randall J. Urban; Weekly Versus Monthly Testosterone Administration on Fast and Slow Skeletal Muscle Fibers in Older Adult Males; J Clin Endocrinol Metab. 2015 Feb; 100(2): E223–E231.

Kawabata F, Mizushige T, Uozumi K, Hayamizu K, Han L, Tsuji T, Kishida T; Fish protein intake induces fast-muscle hypertrophy and reduces liver lipids and serum glucose levels in rats; Biosci Biotechnol Biochem. 2015;

79(1):109-16. Doi: 10.1080/ 09168451. 2014.951025. Epub 2014 Sep 8.

Albers PH, Pedersen AJ, Birk JB, Kristensen DE, Vind BF, Baba O, Nøhr J, Højlund K, Wojtaszewski JF; Human muscle fiber type-specific insulin signaling: impact of obesity and type 2 diabetes; Diabetes. 2015 Feb; 64(2):485-97. Doi: 10.2337/db14-0590. Epub 2014 Sep 3.

Ureczky D, Vácz G, Costa A, Kopper B, Lacza Z, Hortobágyi T, Tihanyi J; The effects of short-term exercise training on peak-torque are time- and fiber-type dependent; J Strength Cond Res. 2014 Aug;28(8):2204-13. Doi: 10.1519/JSC. 0000000000000414.

Ackermann M A, Kontrogianni-Konstantopoulos A. (2011). Myosin binding protein-C slow is a novel substrate for protein kinase A (PKA) and C (PKC) in skeletal muscle. J. Proteome Res., 10, 4547–4555 10,1021/pr200355w

Ackermann M. A., Hu L.-Y. R., Bowman A. L., Bloch R. J., Kontrogianni-Konstantopoulos A. (2009). Obscurin interacts with a novel isoform of MyBP-C slow at the periphery of the sarcomeric M-band and regulates thick filament assembly. Mol. Biol. Cell 20, 2963–2978 10.1091/mbc.E08-12-1251

Rubinow DR, Roca CA, Schmidt PJ, Danaceau MA, Putnam K, Cizza G, et al. Testosterone suppression of CRH-stimulated cortisol in men; Neuropsychopharmacology; 2005; 30:1906–1912.

Per Aagaard; Peter S. Magnusson; Benny Larsson; Michael Kjær; Peter Krustrup; Mechanical Muscle Function, Morphology, and Fiber Type in Lifelong Trained Elderly; Posted 11/16/2007

Ruiz Jonatan R, Sui Xuemei, Felipe Lobelo, Morrow James R, Jackson Allen W, Sjöström Michael, Blair Steven N; Association between muscular strength and mortality in men: prospective cohort study; BMJ. 2008; 337: a439. Published online 2008. Doi: 10.1136/bmj.a439

GENERAL TRAINING ADWISE

Amer Suleman, Kyle D Heffner; Exercise Prescription; Consultant in Electrophysiology and Cardiovascular Medicine, Department of Internal Medicine, Division of Cardiology, Medical City Dallas Hospital. Med. Scape.

Gerber M, Brand S, Elliot C, Holsboer-Trachsler E, Pühse U, Beck J. Aerobic exercise training and burnout: a pilot study with male participants suffering from burnout. BMC Res Notes. 2013a; 6:78.

Garber CE, Blissmer B, Deschenes MR, Franklin BA, Lamonte MJ, Lee IM, Nieman DC, et al. Quantity and quality of exercise for developing and maintaining cardiorespiratory, musculoskeletal, and neuromotor fitness in apparently healthy adults: guidance for prescribing exercise. Med Sci Sports Exerc. 2011;43(7):1334–59.

RESISTANCE TRANING

Fragala MS, Beyer KS, Jajtner AR, Townsend JR, Pruna GJ, Boone CH, et al. Resistance exercise may improve spatial awareness and visual reaction in older adults. J Strength Cond Res. 2014; 28(8):2079–87.http://dx.doi.org/10.1519/JSC.0000000000000520. Doi 10.1519/JSC.0000000000000520

Basso JC, Shang A, Elman M, Karmouta R, Suzuki WA; Acute Exercise Improves Prefrontal Cortex but not Hippocampal Function in Healthy Adults. J Int Neuropsychol Soc. 2015; 2 1(10):791–801. Doi: 10.1017/ S135561771500106X.

Best JR, Chiu BK, Liang Hsu C, Nagamatsu LS, Liu-Ambrose T. Long-Term Effects of Resistance Exercise Training on Cognition and Brain Volume in Older Women: Results from a Randomized Controlled Trial. J Int Neuropsychol Soc. 2015; 21(10):745–56. Doi: 10.1017/S1355617715000673 .

Bossers WJ, van der Woude LH, Boersma F, Hortobagyi T, Scherder EJ, van Heuvelen MJ. A 9-Week Aerobic and Strength Training Program Improves Cognitive and Motor Function in Patients with Dementia: A Randomized, Controlled Trial. Am. J. Geriatric. Psychiatry. 2015. Doi: 10.1016/j.jagp.2014.12.191.

Pedersen BK, Saltin B. Exercise as medicine—evidence for prescribing exercise as therapy in 26 different chronic diseases. Scand J Med Sci Sports. 2015; 25 Suppl 3:1–72. Doi: 10.1111/ sms.12581. [PubMed]

Ruiz JR, Gil-Bea F, Bustamante-Ara N, Rodriguez-Romo G, Fiuza-Luces C, Serra-Rexach JA, et al. Resistance training does not have an effect on cognition or related serum biomarkers in nonagenarians: a randomized controlled trial. Int J Sports Med. 2015; 36(1):54–60. Doi: 10.1055/s-0034-1375693

Ivana Y. Kuo, Barbara E. Ehrlich; Signaling in Muscle Contraction; Cold Spring Harb Perspect Biol; 2015 Feb; 7(2): a006023. Doi: 10.1101/cshperspect.a006023; PMCID: PMC43159 34. PMID: 25646377

Todd Trappe; Influence of aging and long-term unloading on the structure and function of human skeletal muscle; Published in final edited form as; Appl Physiol Nutr

Metab. 2009 Jun; 34(3): 459–464. Doi: 10,1139/h09-041; PMCID: PMC3056056. NIHMSID: NIHMS27716

TYPE 1 MUSCLES AND DEACTIVATION

http://www.stretching-exercises-guide.com/back-stretches.html

Nelson AG1, Kokkonen J, Arnall DA; Twenty minutes of passive stretching lowers glucose levels in an at-risk population: an experimental study; J Physiother. 2011; 57(3):173-8. Doi: 10.1016/S1836-9553(11)70038-8.

Manoel ME, Harris-Love MO, Danoff JV, Miller TA; Acute effects of static, dynamic, and proprioceptive neuromuscular facilitation stretching on muscle power in women; J Strength Cond Res. Sep 2008;22(5):1528–1534 [PubMed]

Kistler BM, Walsh MS, Horn TS, Cox RH; The acute effects of static stretching on the sprint performance of collegiate men in the 60- and 100-m dash after a dynamic warm-up; J Strength Cond Res. 2010 Sep;24(9):2280-4. Doi: 10.1519/JSC. 0b013e3181e58dd7.

Curry BS, Chengkalath D, Crouch GJ, Romance M, Manns PJ; Acute effects of dynamic stretching, static stretching, and light aerobic activity on muscular performance in women. J Strength Cond Res. Sep 2009; 23(6):1811–1819

Torres EM, Kraemer WJ, Vingren JL; Effects of stretching on upper-body muscular performance; J Strength Cond Res. Jul 2008; 22(4):1279–1285.

Yamaguchi T, Ishii K; Effects of static stretching for 30 seconds and dynamic stretching on leg extension power; J Strength Cond Res. Aug 2005; 19(3):677–683

Kay AD, et al Blazevich AJ. Concentric muscle contractions before static stretching minimize, but do not remove, stretch-induced force deficits. J Appl Physiol. Mar 2010;108(3):637–645

Power K, Behm D, Cahill F, Carroll M, Young W. An acute bout of static stretching: effects on force and jumping performance. Med Sci Sports Exerc. Aug 2004;36(8):13891396.

Robbins JW, Scheuermann BW; Varierande mängder akut statisk stretching och dess effekt på vertikal hoppprestanda; J Strength Cond Res. Maj 2008; 22 (3): 781-786.

Taylor DC, Dalton JD Jr, Seaber AV, Garrett WE Jr; Viscoelastic properties of muscle-tendons units. The biomechanical effects of stretching; Am J Sports Med. 1990 May-Jun; 18 (3):300-9.

Caplan N, Rogers R, Parr MK, Hayes PR; The effect of proprioceptive neuromuscular facilitation and static stretch training on running mechanics; J Strength Cond Res. Jul 2009;23(4):1175–1180

Small K, Mc NL, Matthews M; A systematic review into the efficacy of static stretching as part of a warm-up for the prevention of exercise-related injury; Res Sports Med. Jul 2008; 16(3):213–231.

Ben M, Harvey LA; Regular stretch does not increase muscle extensibility: a randomized controlled trial; Scandinavian journal of medicine & science in sports. Feb 2010; 20(1):136–144

O'Sullivan K, Murray E, Sainsbury D. Effekten av uppvärmning, statisk stretching och dynamisk tretching på flexibiliteten hos tidigare skadade personer. BMC Musculoskelet Disord. 2009; 10: 37.

Dalrymple KJ, Davis SE, Dwyer GB, Moir GL; Effect of static and dynamic stretching on vertical jump performance in collegiate women volleyball players; J Strength Cond Res. 2010 Jan;24(1):149-55. Doi: 10.1519/JSC.0b013e3181b29614. PMID: 20042927

de Weijer VC, Gorniak GC, Shamus E; The effect of static stretch and warm-up exercise on hamstring length over the course of 24 hours; J Orthop Sports Phys Ther. Dec 2003; 33(12):727–733 [PubMed]

Marek SM, Cramer JT, Fincher AL, Massey LL, Dangelmaier SM, Purkayastha S, Fitz KA, Culbertson JY; Acute Effects of Static and Proprioceptive Neuromuscular

Reid DA, McNair PJ; Effect of an acute hamstring stretch in people with and without osteoarthritis of the knee; Physio-therapy. 2010 Mar; 96(1):14-21. Doi: 10.1016/j.physio. 2009. 06.010. Epub 2009 Sep 4; J Athl. Train; 2005 Jun; 40(2):94-103.

RESTLESS LEGS SYNDROME

Chiara Cirelli; The genetic and molecular regulation of sleep: from fruit flies to humans; Nat Rev Neurosci. 2009 Aug; 10(8): 549–560. doi: 10.1038/nrn2683. PMCID: PMC2767184. NIHMSID: NIHMS152790. PMID: 19617891

Melissa McManama Aukerman, MS; Douglas Aukerman, MD; Max Bayard, MD; Fred Tudiver, MD; Lydia Thorp, MD; Beth Bailey; Exercise and Restless Legs Syndrome: A Randomized. Medscape Newes; Posted 10-20-2006.

Jens P. Reese; Karin Stiasny-Kolster; Wolfgang H. Oertel; Richard C. Dodel; Health-related Quality of Life and Economic Burden in Patients With Restless Legs Syndrome; Posted 11/28/2007. Medscape News.

Mario Giovanni Terzano; Liborio Parrino; Enrica Bonanni; Fabio Cirignotta; Franco Ferrillo; Gian Luigi Gigli; Mariantonietta Savarese; Luigi Ferini-Strambi; Insomnia in General Practice; A Consensus Report Produced by Sleep Specialists and Primary-Care Physicians in Italy; Posted 12/22/2005

Phil Page; Current concept in muscle stretching for exercise and rehabilititation; Int J Sports Phys Ther. 2012 Feb; 7(1): 109–119; PMCID: PMC3273886

McHugh MP, Magnusson SP, Gleim GW, Nicholas JA; Viscoelastic stress relaxation in human skeletal muscle; Med Sci Sports Exerc. 1992 Dec; 24(12):1375-82

Printed in the United States
By Bookmasters